HEALTH CARE ISSUES, COSTS AND ACCESS

MEDICARE SPENDING AND THE INDEPENDENT PAYMENT ADVISORY BOARD

HEALTH CARE ISSUES, COSTS AND ACCESS

Additional books in this series can be found on Nova's website under the Series tab.

Additional E-books in this series can be found on Nova's website under the e-books tab.

PUBLIC HEALTH IN THE 21ST CENTURY

Additional books in this series can be found on Nova's website under the Series tab.

Additional E-books in this series can be found on Nova's website under the e-books tab.

HEALTH CARE ISSUES, COSTS AND ACCESS

MEDICARE SPENDING AND THE INDEPENDENT PAYMENT ADVISORY BOARD

RYAN D. BROWN
AND
STEVEN J. MARTIN
EDITORS

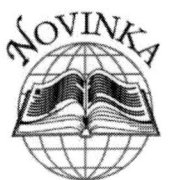

Nova Science Publishers, Inc.
New York

Copyright © 2012 by Nova Science Publishers, Inc.

All rights reserved. No part of this book may be reproduced, stored in a retrieval system or transmitted in any form or by any means: electronic, electrostatic, magnetic, tape, mechanical photocopying, recording or otherwise without the written permission of the Publisher.

For permission to use material from this book please contact us:
Telephone 631-231-7269; Fax 631-231-8175
Web Site: http://www.novapublishers.com

NOTICE TO THE READER

The Publisher has taken reasonable care in the preparation of this book, but makes no expressed or implied warranty of any kind and assumes no responsibility for any errors or omissions. No liability is assumed for incidental or consequential damages in connection with or arising out of information contained in this book. The Publisher shall not be liable for any special, consequential, or exemplary damages resulting, in whole or in part, from the readers' use of, or reliance upon, this material. Any parts of this book based on government reports are so indicated and copyright is claimed for those parts to the extent applicable to compilations of such works.

Independent verification should be sought for any data, advice or recommendations contained in this book. In addition, no responsibility is assumed by the publisher for any injury and/or damage to persons or property arising from any methods, products, instructions, ideas or otherwise contained in this publication.

This publication is designed to provide accurate and authoritative information with regard to the subject matter covered herein. It is sold with the clear understanding that the Publisher is not engaged in rendering legal or any other professional services. If legal or any other expert assistance is required, the services of a competent person should be sought. FROM A DECLARATION OF PARTICIPANTS JOINTLY ADOPTED BY A COMMITTEE OF THE AMERICAN BAR ASSOCIATION AND A COMMITTEE OF PUBLISHERS.

Additional color graphics may be available in the e-book version of this book.

Library of Congress Cataloging-in-Publication Data

ISBN: 978-1-62081-112-2

Published by Nova Science Publishers, Inc. † New York

CONTENTS

Preface		vii
Chapter 1	The Independent Payment Advisory Board *David Newman and Christopher M. Davis*	1
Chapter 2	PPACA: A Brief Overview of the Law, Implementation, and Legal Challenges *Hinda Chaikind, Curtis W. Copeland, C. Stephen Redhead and Jennifer Staman*	47
Index		57

PREFACE

Among some proponents of health care reform, a major impetus for reform, in additional to improving quality and increasing access, has been the rising cost of the Medicare program. In response, in part, to overall growth in Medicare program expenditures and growth in expenditures per Medicare beneficiary, the Patient Protection and Affordable Care Act (PPACA), created the Independent Payment Advisory Board (IPAB), and charged the Board with developing proposals to "reduce the per capita rate of growth in Medicare spending." This book provides an overview of the Board's structure, and reviews the expedited and other parliamentary procedures that relate to congressional consideration of the Board's proposals and impact.

Chapter 1- In response, in part, to overall growth in Medicare program expenditures and growth in expenditures per Medicare beneficiary, the Patient Protection and Affordable Care Act (PPACA, P.L. 111-148, as amended) created the Independent Payment Advisory Board (IPAB, or the Board) and charged the Board with developing proposals to "reduce the per capita rate of growth in Medicare spending." The Secretary of Health and Human Services (the Secretary) is directed to implement the Board's proposals automatically unless Congress affirmatively acts to alter the Board's proposals or to discontinue the automatic implementation of such proposals.

The annual IPAB sequence of events begins each year, starting April 30, 2013, with the Chief Actuary of the Centers for Medicare & Medicaid Services calculating a Medicare per capita growth rate and a Medicare per capita target growth rate. If the Chief Actuary determines that the Medicare per capita growth rate exceeds the Medicare per capita target growth rate, the Chief Actuary would establish an applicable savings target—the amount by which the Board must reduce future spending. This determination by the Chief

Actuary also triggers a requirement that the Board prepare a proposal to reduce the growth in the Medicare per capita growth rate by the applicable savings target. The Board cannot ration care, raise premiums, increase cost sharing, or otherwise restrict benefits or modify eligibility. In generating its proposals, the Board is directed to consider, among other things, Medicare solvency, quality and access to care, the effects of changes in payments to providers, and those dually eligible for Medicare and Medicaid. If the Board fails to act, the Secretary is directed to prepare a proposal.

Chapter 2- In March 2010, the 111th Congress passed health reform legislation, the Patient Protection and Affordable Care Act (P.L. 111-148), as amended by the Health Care and Education Reconciliation Act of 2010 (P.L. 111-152). Jointly referred to as PPACA, the law increases access to health insurance coverage, expands federal private health insurance market requirements, and requires the creation of health insurance exchanges to provide individuals and small employers with access to insurance. The costs for expanding access to health insurance and other provisions are projected to be offset by increased taxes and revenues and reduced Medicare and Medicaid spending. Implementation of PPACA, which is scheduled to unfold over the next few years, involves all the major health care stakeholders, including the federal and state governments, as well as employers, insurers, and health care providers. Following the enactment of PPACA, state attorneys general and others have brought a number of lawsuits challenging provisions of PPACA, including the individual mandate, on constitutional grounds.

This report provides a brief summary of major PPACA provisions, implementation and oversight activities, and current legal challenges.

In: Medicare Spending and the Independent ...   ISBN: 978-1- 62081-112-2
Editors: R. D. Brown and S. J. Martin   © 2012 Nova Science Publishers, Inc.

Chapter 1

THE INDEPENDENT PAYMENT ADVISORY BOARD[*]

David Newman and Christopher M. Davis

SUMMARY

In response, in part, to overall growth in Medicare program expenditures and growth in expenditures per Medicare beneficiary, the Patient Protection and Affordable Care Act (PPACA, P.L. 111-148, as amended) created the Independent Payment Advisory Board (IPAB, or the Board) and charged the Board with developing proposals to "reduce the per capita rate of growth in Medicare spending." The Secretary of Health and Human Services (the Secretary) is directed to implement the Board's proposals automatically unless Congress affirmatively acts to alter the Board's proposals or to discontinue the automatic implementation of such proposals.

The annual IPAB sequence of events begins each year, starting April 30, 2013, with the Chief Actuary of the Centers for Medicare & Medicaid Services calculating a Medicare per capita growth rate and a Medicare per capita target growth rate. If the Chief Actuary determines that the Medicare per capita growth rate exceeds the Medicare per capita target growth rate, the Chief Actuary would establish an applicable savings target—the amount by which the Board must reduce future spending. This determination by the Chief

---

[*] This is an edited, reformatted and augmented version of a Congressional Research Service publication, CRS Report for Congress R41511, dated April 18, 2011.

Actuary also triggers a requirement that the Board prepare a proposal to reduce the growth in the Medicare per capita growth rate by the applicable savings target. The Board cannot ration care, raise premiums, increase cost sharing, or otherwise restrict benefits or modify eligibility. In generating its proposals, the Board is directed to consider, among other things, Medicare solvency, quality and access to care, the effects of changes in payments to providers, and those dually eligible for Medicare and Medicaid. If the Board fails to act, the Secretary is directed to prepare a proposal.

Board proposals must be submitted to the Secretary by September 1 of each year and to the President and Congress by January 15 of the following year. Board proposals are "fast-tracked" in Congress, and IPAB proposals go into force automatically unless Congress affirmatively acts to amend or block them within a stated period of time and under circumstances specified in the Act. Section 3403(d) of the Act establishes special "fast track" parliamentary procedures governing House and Senate committee consideration, and Senate floor consideration, of legislation implementing the Board or Secretary's proposal. These procedures differ from the parliamentary mechanisms the chambers usually use to consider most legislation and are designed to ensure that Congress can act promptly on the implementing legislation should it choose to do so. PPACA also established a second "fast track" parliamentary mechanism for consideration of legislation discontinuing the automatic implementation process for the recommendations of the Board.

The Board's charge is to develop proposals for the Secretary to implement that reduce the per capita growth in Medicare expenditures, not to reduce Medicare expenditures. Therefore, while the Congressional Budget Office projects that the cumulative impact of the Board's recommendations from 2015 through 2019 will reduce total spending by $15.5 billion, during the same period, Medicare expenditures will total $3.9 trillion with average spending per beneficiary forecast to increase from $13,374 to $15,749. While the Board's potential impact on total expenditures is likely to be relatively small compared to overall Medicare expenditures, its impact on particular Medicare providers or suppliers may be significant, particularly if the Board alters payment mechanisms. Finally, the Board's impact may be larger if private insurers continue to track Medicare payment policies and adopt similar reductions in payments to their providers and suppliers.

INTRODUCTION

The Patient Protection and Affordable Care Act (PPACA, P.L. 111-148, as amended) created the Independent Payment Advisory Board (IPAB, or the Board) to "reduce the per capita rate of growth in Medicare spending."[1] The Board's proposals will be implemented by the Secretary of Health and Human Services (the Secretary) unless Congress acts either by formulating its own proposal to achieve the same savings or by discontinuing the automatic implementation process defined in the statute.

This report, which provides an overview of the Board, begins with a discussion of the rationale behind the creation of an independent Medicare board and briefly reviews prior proposals for similar boards and commissions. The report then describes the structure of the Board, the calculations and determinations required to be made by the Office of the Chief Actuary (the Chief Actuary) in the Centers for Medicare & Medicaid Services (CMS) that trigger a Board proposal, and the content of and constraints on Board proposals—including the Medicare productivity exemptions under § 3401 of PPACA. In addition, the report reviews the expedited and other parliamentary procedures that relate to congressional consideration of Board proposals and other Board-related activities, and concludes with a description of how the Board's proposals are to be implemented and their possible impact. **Appendix A** details key dates for IPAB implementation and various reports required by the law, and **Appendix B** compares the IPAB with the Medicare Payment Advisory Commission (MedPAC). **Appendix C** summarizes the Medicare productivity exemptions in § 3401 of PPACA as they relate to § 3403.

BACKGROUND

Among some proponents of health care reform, a major impetus for reform, in addition to improving quality and increasing access, has been the rising cost of the Medicare program.

Medical Inflation

For the past 25 years, annual medical inflation has exceeded annual overall inflation in every year but one (see **Figure 1**).[2] Specifically, over this time period, medical inflation has on average been roughly 2.2 percentage points higher each year than overall inflation. Moreover, Medicare spending during this same period has increased 8.5% per year, while total federal outlays during this same period increased by only 5.3% per year.[3] While some of the growth in Medicare expenditures can be attributed to the increase in the number of Medicare beneficiaries, Medicare per enrollee expenditures rose 6.3% per year from 1985 through 2008—faster than overall medical inflation.[4] Had spending per Medicare beneficiary increased at just the rate of overall inflation over the 1985 through 2008 period, per enrollee expenditures in 2008 would have been slightly less than $4,600 as compared to actual 2008 Medicare Part A and Part B expenditures of $9,448 per beneficiary.[5]

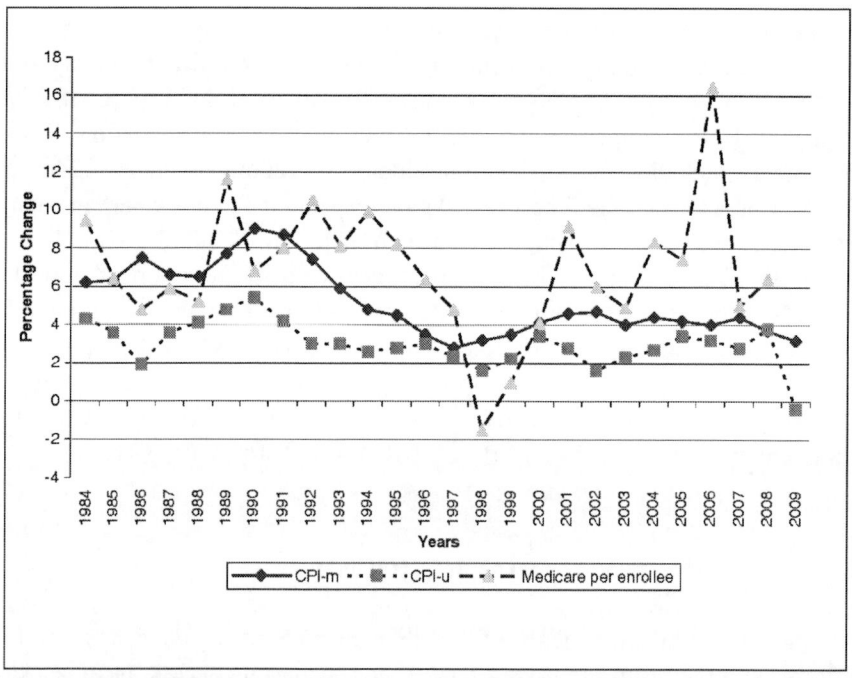

Source: CRS analysis of data from U.S. Department of Labor, Bureau of Labor Statistics, http://data.bls.gov; http://www.cms.gov/ National Health Expend Data/downloads/tables.pdf, Table 13.

Notes: CPI_u refers the Consumer Price Index for all items and services and CPI_m refers to the Consumer Price Index for medical inflation.

Figure 1. Annual Change in CPI_u, CPI_m and Per Enrollee Medicare Expenditures.

Again, the legislation's stated goal of the Board is to reduce the per capita *growth* in Medicare expenditures, not to reduce *overall* Medicare expenditures. The Board achieves this goal by developing proposals for the Secretary to implement that reduce the growth in Medicare expenditures. Therefore, while the Congressional Budget Office (CBO) projects that the cumulative impact of the Board's recommendations from 2015 through 2019 will reduce total spending by $15.5 billion, during the same period total Medicare expenditures are projected to be $3.9 trillion with average spending per beneficiary increasing from $13,374 in 2015 to $15,749 in 2019.[6] These savings represent a reduction of about $60.00 per year per Medicare beneficiary over the 2015 through 2019 period.

Earlier Medicare Reform Proposals

Since these historic patterns of growth in overall health care spending, and Medicare in particular, are viewed as not being sustainable,[7] several proposals have been advanced over the years to create an independent policy-making entity that would be charged with limiting the future growth in Medicare expenditures;[8] be insulated from special interests and lobbyists since these entities would be appointed, rather than elected, and serve for extended terms; and such officials would be able to make the so-called "hard decisions" to control rising costs. Moreover, it has been assumed that these entities would possess the specialized expertise needed to make operational decisions regarding payments and focus initiatives on beneficiary interests and the longer term financial viability of the program.

For instance, in 2000 and 2001 Senators Breaux and Frist introduced reform proposals to increase CMS's budget, create separate agencies to administer parts of the program, and establish a Medicare Board to manage competition among private plans and traditional Medicare (referred to as "Breaux-Frist I," S. 1895, and "Breaux-Frist II," S. 358).

Interest in an independent health care entity reemerged during early discussions of what became PPACA. Former Senator Tom Daschle proposed the Federal Health Board, modeled after the Federal Reserve Board, with broad authority over both private and public health care programs, including benefit and coverage recommendations, regulation of private insurance markets, and improvements in quality of care.[9]

In June 2009, Senator Rockefeller introduced the Medicare Payment Advisory Commission (MedPAC) Reform Act of 2009 (S. 1380 in the 111th

Congress), which would have altered MedPAC from its current 15-member advisory commission to an 11-member executive branch agency with authority to make both payment and coverage decisions (see **Appendix B** for a sideby-side comparison of MedPAC and IPAB). In order to achieve program savings, the Commission was directed "to implement payment policies, methodologies, and rates and coverage policies and methodologies ... estimated to reduce expenditures under this title by not less than 1.5 percent annually."

In July 2009, the President submitted a draft proposal to Congress titled the Independent Medicare Advisory Council Act of 2009 (referred to as the IMAC proposal). This proposal would have established a five-member council to advise the President on Medicare payment rates for certain providers. While the council would have had authority to recommend broader policy reforms, its authority outside of Medicare payment policy was limited.

Finally, during the recent health care reform deliberations, the Senate Finance Committee included a provision (§ 3403) to establish an independent Medicare advisory board in the now enacted PPACA. Section 10320, added by the manager's amendment, broadened the scope of the Board to make recommendations to slow the growth in non-federal programs and changed the name of the entity to the Independent Payment Advisory Board, to reflect these additional responsibilities.

The perceived merits to some of an independent board are the perceived shortcomings to others. For instance, as Medicare expenditures represent a sizable proportion of federal outlays, approximately 13% in FY2010, for some critics such a large proportion of expenditures should not be beyond the scrutiny and review of elected officials or the public. Second, there is concern that boards, such as IPAB, are singularly focused on reducing spending, that tradeoffs exist between spending and quality, and that these tradeoffs are best dealt with by elected officials. Finally, similar efforts to "automatically" control health care spending, such as the sustainable growth rate formula, used to update Medicare physician payments, potentially demonstrate that such supposedly automatic mechanisms do not effectively remove special interests or Congress from the process.[10] For proponents, removing short term political and public opinion, focusing on spending, and using automatic mechanisms is required to reduce the growth in expenditures and rationalize health care decision making.

STRUCTURE AND OPERATIONS OF IPAB

The explicit charge given by PPACA to the Board in § 3403(b) is to "reduce the per capita rate of growth in Medicare expenditures." As described in more detail below, beginning in 2013, and each subsequent year, the Chief Actuary needs to calculate the *Medicare per capita growth rate*— the five-year average growth in Medicare program spending per enrollee and the *Medicare per capita target growth rate*—the rate Medicare expenditures would grow without triggering interventions under this section. If the Chief Actuary determines that projected five-year per capita growth rate in Medicare expenditures two years hence exceeds the projected per capita target growth rate, the Chief Actuary needs to establish an applicable savings target—the amount by which the Board must reduce future spending. The Chief Actuary's determination also triggers a requirement that the Board prepare a proposal to reduce Medicare expenditures by an amount at least equal to the applicable savings target.

While funding for the Board is authorized beginning in FY2012 and the Chief Actuary makes its first determination in 2013, the statute does not provide a date by which the Board is to begin its operations. Below, the Board's membership, structure, and budget are described.

Membership

The Board will be composed of 15 members appointed by the President with the advice and consent of the Senate.[11] As such, the members are officers of the United States under the appointments clause of the U.S. Constitution.[12] The Secretary of Health and Human Services, the Administrator of CMS, and the Administrator of the Health Resources and Services Administration are ex-officio nonvoting members. In selecting individuals for nomination, the President is to consult with the majority and minority leadership of the Senate and House of Representatives—each respectively, regarding the appointment of three members. The Chairperson is appointed by the President, with the advice and consent of the Senate, from among the members of the Board.

Qualifications of Board Members

The appointed members of the Board are to provide varied professional and geographic representation and possess recognized expertise in

- health finance and economics,
- actuarial science,
- health facility management,
- health plans and integrated delivery systems, and
- reimbursement of health facilities.

In addition, the board members are to be drawn from a wide range of backgrounds, including but not limited to

- physicians (allopathic and osteopathic) and other health professionals, providers of health services, and related fields;
- experts in the area of pharmaco-economics or prescription drug benefit programs;
- employers;
- third-party payers; and
- individuals skilled in the conduct and interpretation of biomedical health services, and health economics research and expertise in outcomes and effectiveness research and technology assessment.

Members should also include representatives of consumers and the elderly. A majority of the appointed members cannot be individuals directly involved in the provision or management of the delivery of Medicare items and services.

Term of Office

With exceptions for initial Board members and those appointed to fill a vacancy with an unexpired term, each appointed member may serve two consecutive six year terms.[13] If appointed to fill a vacancy, the member can serve two additional consecutive terms. Appointments to initially fill the Board are staggered with terms of one, three, or six years.

Conditions of Service

Appointed members of the Board will be subject to financial and conflict of interest disclosures and will be treated as officers in the executive branch for purposes of the Ethics in Government Act of 1978.[14] Moreover, there is a blanket prohibition against appointed members engaging in any other business, vocation, or employment. In addition, former members of the Board will be precluded for one year from lobbying before the Board, the Department of Health and Human Services, or any of the relevant committees of jurisdiction of Congress.[15] Finally, appointed members of the Board may be removed by the President only for neglect of duty or malfeasance in office.[16]

Compensation

Appointed members of the Board will be compensated at a rate equal to Level III of the Executive Schedule ($165,300 for 2011), and the Chairperson will be compensated at a rate equal to Level II ($179,700 for 2011).

The Board's Structure, Staff and Budget

The Chairperson will be the principal executive officer of the Board and supervise employees. The Board will elect its own vice Chairperson to act in the absence or disability of the Chairperson or in the event of a vacancy. In addition, the law provides that the Board can hire an executive director and a staff—either detailed from other Federal agencies or direct hires—to perform its duties.

The budget for the Board for FY2012 is $15 million, with annual adjustments based on increases in the consumer price index (CPI)—only slightly more than the MedPAC budget. The Board will be funded out of the Medicare trust funds—specifically, 60% of the Board's funds will come from the Federal Hospital Insurance Trust Fund and 40% from the Federal Supplementary Medical Insurance Trust Fund.

Table 1. Three-Year Sequence of Events

Determination Year (DY)	
By April 30	Chief Actuary of CMS makes projections and determination
By September 1	Draft proposal sent by IPAB to MedPAC for consultation Draft proposal sent by IPAB to Secretary for review and comment
Proposal Year (PY)	
By January 15	Proposal submitted by IPAB to Congress and the President
By January 25	Secretary submits own proposal to Congress and the President, with a copy to MedPAC, if IPAB was required to submit a proposal but failed to do so
By March 1	Secretary submits report containing review and comments to Congress on IPAB proposal (unless the Secretary submitted own proposal because IPAB failed to do so)
By April 1	Deadline for specified Congressional Committees to consider the submitted proposal and report out legislative language implementing the recommendations. Congress has the authority to develop its own proposal provided it meets the same fiscal requirements as established for the Board and meets this deadline.
Beginning August 15	Secretary implements the proposal subject to exceptions
On October 1	Recommendations relating to fiscal year payment rate changes take effect
Implementation Year (IY)	
On January 1	Recommendations relating to Medicare Part C and D payments take effect Recommendations relating to calendar year payment rate changes take effect

Source: CRS analysis of P.L. 111-148, as amended.

THE DETERMINATION PROCESS

This section describes the role of the Chief Actuary and the determination process by which the Chief Actuary establishes whether the projected per capita Medicare expenditures will exceed certain target levels. The Chief Actuary's determination sets in motion a three-year sequence of events (see

Table 1). In addition, this section describes the key calculations that the Chief Actuary will need to make beginning in 2013 and provides an illustrative example of these calculations.

The three-year sequence begins each year with the Chief Actuary making a determination, by April 30, as to whether the projected per capita Medicare expenditures will exceed certain target levels. The year in which the Chief Actuary makes its determination is referred to as the determination year (DY). The next year is referred to as the proposal year (PY) and the following year is the implementation year (IY).

Key Calculations by the Chief Actuary

Beginning in 2013, the Chief Actuary is required to determine several key calculations, based on an analysis of a five-year period. The DY is the midpoint of the five-year period, as shown in **Figure 2**.

The Chief Actuary is required to calculate

- the Medicare per capita growth rate (the "growth rate"), and
- the Medicare per capita target growth rate (the "target growth rate").

The *growth rate* is defined as the projected five-year average (using the DY as the midpoint of the five years) growth in Medicare program spending per enrollee. *Medicare program spending* includes spending for Medicare Parts A, B, and D, net of premiums.[17] For example, for the 2013 DY, the Chief Actuary will use the growth in spending for 2011-2015.

Using the same five-year period, the *target growth rate* will initially be calculated based on the midpoint between the five-year average overall inflation (using the Consumer Price Index for all items and services, the CPI_u) and five-year average medical inflation (using the Consumer Price Index for medical inflation, the CPI_m). However, beginning with the 2018 DY, the *target growth rate* will be tied to the growth of the economy, based on the five-year average increase in the nominal Gross Domestic Product (GDP) plus one percentage point.

For DYs prior to 2018, the *target growth rate* is determined as follows:

- Calculate the percent increase in each year for both the CPI_u and the CPI_m.

- Add the CPI_u and CPI_m together for each year and take the simple average by dividing by 2.
- Using the simple average for each year, calculate the average annualized rate of growth for the entire five-year period.
- The average annualized rate of growth is a single number, which is the *target growth rate* for the five-year period.

For DYs beginning in 2018, the *target growth rate* will be the projected five-year average percentage increase in the nominal GDP per capita plus one percentage point. Using this formula will constrain future increases in Medicare expenditures more closely to the rate of growth in the economy. However because the formula adds one percentage point each year to the increase in nominal GDP, Medicare expenditures could continue to grow more quickly than the economy.

If the Chief Actuary finds that the *growth rate* does not exceed the *targeted growth rate*, the process for the year ends. If the Chief Actuary determines that the *growth rate* exceeds the *target growth rate* for any DY, the Chief Actuary is required to establish an *applicable savings target* for the IY. The *applicable savings target* is an amount equal to the product of the total projected Medicare expenditures in the PY times the *applicable percent*. The *applicable percent* is defined as the lesser of either the projected excess for the IY (the amount by which Medicare spending is forecast to exceed the targeted growth in spending expressed as a percent of total Medicare expenditures) or the percent as specified in the statute (0.5% in IY 2015; 1.0% in IY 2016; 1.25% in IY 2017; and 1.5% in 2018 and any subsequent IY). In either event, the percent is converted to a dollar amount by which Medicare program expenditures must be reduced.

For example, if the Chief Actuary determines in 2013 that the *growth rate* will exceed the *target growth rate* by 0.75% for IY 2015, the Board would need to make recommendations that reduce overall Medicare expenditures by 0.5 0% (the *applicable percent* for IY20 15). Alternatively, if the Chief Actuary determines in 2013 that the *growth rate* exceeds the *target growth rate* by the projected excess, 0.35% for IY20 15, the Board would need to make recommendations that reduce overall Medicare expenditures by 0.35%. (See **Table 2** for the annual *applicable percent* and other changes in key terms over time.)

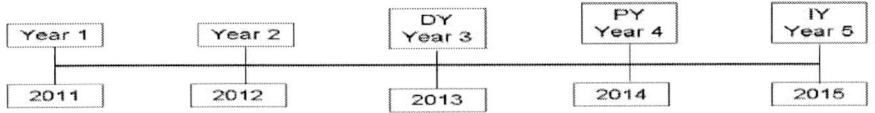

Figure 2. Initial Five-Year Sequence Determination Year 2013.

Table 2. Definition and Applicability of Key Terms Over Time

Key Terms	DY 2013 PY 2014 IY 2015	DY 2014 PY 2015 IY 2016	DY 2015 PY 2016 IY 2017	DY 2016 PY 2017 IY 2018	DY 2017 PY 2018 IY 2019	DY 2018+ PY 2019+ IY 2020+
Medicare Per Capita Growth Rate	The projected five-year average (the projected implementation year and four prior years) of the growth in Medicare program spending per unduplicated enrollee.					
Medicare Per Capita Target Growth Rate	The projected five-year average (the projected implementation year and four prior years) percentage increase in the average of the projected percentage increase (if any) in the Consumer Price Index for All Urban Consumers (all items, U.S. city average) and the Consumer Price Index for All Urban Consumers (medical care, U.S. city average).					The projected five-year average percentage increase in nominal GDP per capita ending in the IY plus one percentage point, for each of 5 years
Applicable Percent (if growth rate exceeds target growth rate)	The lesser of 0.5 percent or the projected excess	The lesser of 1.0 percent or the projected excess	The lesser of 1.25 percent or the projected excess	The lesser of 1.5 percent or the projected excess	The lesser of 1.5 percent or the projected excess	The lesser of 1.5 percent or the projected excess
Applicable Savings Target	The product of the total projected Medicare expenditures in the proposal year and the *applicable percent* for that implementation year.					

DY = Determination Year; PY = Proposal Year; IY = Implementation Year.
Source: CRS analysis of P.L. 111-148, as amended.

A Hypothetical Example

This section provides an example to illustrate the calculations the Chief Actuary needs to develop, beginning April 2013 and each year thereafter, that form the basis of the Chief Actuary's determination (see **Table 3**). For this example, Year 1 is the first year of data included in the calculation, Year 3 is the DY, Year 4 is the PY, and Year 5 is the IY. It is further assumed that the *applicable percent* is 0.50% and that total projected Medicare expenditures in the PY are $600 billion.

First, in April of Year 3, the Chief Actuary must calculate the *growth rate*—the projected five-year average growth in per capita Medicare spending (Column A) over the five-year period ending with the IY.[18] In addition, the Chief Actuary must calculate the *target growth rate*. For the current DY, Year 3, this is the projected five-year average percentage increase in the average of the projected increase in the CPI_u and the CPI_m, also beginning with Year 1 and ending with the IY. Column B presents the annual percentage change in the CPI_u, ending with Year 5, the IY, and column C presents the annual percentage change in the CPI_m ending in Year 5. Column D provides the annual average percentage change in the CPI_u and CPI_m and the five-year annual growth in the average, ending in Year 5.[19] As the Chief Actuary makes these calculations in the DY for an IY two years hence, some of the data the Chief Actuary will rely on will be projections.

Continuing the example, since the average annualized five-year *per capita growth rate* of 4.99% exceeds the five-year average annualized *target growth rate* of 3.32%, the Chief Actuary must establish an *applicable savings target* for the IY. The *applicable savings target* is calculated by multiplying the projected Medicare program spending in the PY by the lesser of

- the *applicable percent* for the IY (in this example, 0.5%), or
- the difference in columns A and D (column E).

Since 0.5% is less than 1.67%, 0.5% would be used. Therefore, the *applicable savings target* is $600 billion multiplied by 0.005, or $3 billion.[20]

In summary, in this hypothetical example, the Chief Actuary's calculations determined that the *growth rate* exceeded the *target growth rate*. Given this determination, the Chief Actuary calculated the *applicable savings target*, which required the Board to prepare a proposal that reduces Medicare expenditures by the *applicable savings target*.

Table 3. Example for Hypothetical Implementation Year

Year	(A) Annual Percentage Growth in Per Capita Medicare Spending	(B) Annual Percentage Change in CPI_u	(C) Annual Percentage Change in CPI_m	(D) Average of CPI_u and CPI_m	(E) Projected Excess[a]
Year 1	1.00%	2.20%	3.5%	2.85%	
Year 2	4.10%	3.40%	4.10%	3.75%	
DY (Year 3)	9.10%	2.80%	4.60%	3.70%	
PY (Year 4)	6.00%	1.60%	4.70%	3.15%	
IY (Year 5)	4.90%	2.30%	4.00%	3.15%	
Five-year Average Annualized Growth Rate	4.99%			3.32%	1.67%

Source: CRS analysis of P.L. 111-148, as amended.

a. The projected excess is the difference in five-year average in column (A) and column (D)

Activating the Trigger

The Chief Actuary applied this calculation to historic data to better understand the potential impact on Medicare spending. The Chief Actuary reported that "actual Medicare cost growth per beneficiary was below the target level in only four of the last 25 years, with three of those years immediately following the Balanced Budget Act of 1997."[21] Thus, in most recent years past, depending on the target growth rate and assuming no other changes, the Chief Actuary would have made a determination that triggered a Board proposal. The assumption of no other changes, however, may not be realistic since it assumes that any Board's recommendations implemented in prior years had no lasting effect on costs in later years and at the same time ignores the impact of other statutory and regulatory changes that potentially affected the Medicare program.

THE IPAB MEDICARE PROPOSAL PROCESS

If the Chief Actuary makes a determination by April 30 of the DY that the *growth rate* for an IY is forecast to exceed the *target growth rate* for that year, the Board is to develop a detailed proposal to reduce the *growth rate* by the *applicable savings target*. This section details the proposal process and key elements of Board proposals.

Proposal Schedule

By September 1 of each DY, the Board submits a draft of its proposal for review to the Secretary and to MedPAC for consultation. The Board transmits its annual proposal to Congress and the President on January 15 of each PY, beginning 2014. By March 1 of each PY, the Secretary submits comments to Congress on Board proposals.

If the Board is required to develop a proposal but fails to transmit its proposal to Congress and the President by January 15 of any PY, the Secretary is required to develop a proposal and transmit it to Congress and the President, with a copy to MedPAC, by January 25 of the PY. The statute does not define a specific role for MedPAC after it receives the proposal.

Scope of Proposals

PPACA directs the Board that its proposal

- relate only to the Medicare program;
- result in a net reduction in total Medicare program expenditures in the IY that are at least equal to the *applicable savings target* established by the Chief Actuary;
- not include any recommendation to ration care, raise revenues or Medicare beneficiary premiums, increase cost-sharing, restrict benefits, or alter eligibility;
- not reduce payments to providers or suppliers scheduled to receive a reduction in payment as the result of productivity adjustments under § 3401 (see **Appendix C**);

- include, as appropriate, recommendations to reduce Medicare payments under parts C and D, such as reductions in direct subsidy payments to Medicare Advantage and prescription drug plans[22] that are related to administrative expenses (including profits) for basic coverage, denying high bids or removing high bids for prescription drug coverage from the calculation of the national average monthly bid amount[23] and reductions in payments to Medicare Advantage plans that are related to administrative expenses (including profits) and performance bonuses for Medicare Advantage plans;[24] and
- include recommendations with respect to administrative funding for the Secretary to carry out the Board's recommendations.

In addition, if the Chief Actuary has made a determination that the growth in per capita national health expenditures is greater than the Medicare per capita growth rate (a determination first made in 2018), then the Board's proposals should be designed to help reduce the growth in national health expenditures while maintaining or enhancing Medicare beneficiary access to quality care.

In order to develop proposals, the Board is empowered to request and receive official data. In addition, the Board has the power to hold hearings, including field hearings, and to take testimony, and receive evidence as the Board considers advisable. Finally, Board proposals require a majority vote of the appointed members.

Additional Considerations

In developing its proposal, the Board is also directed, to the extent feasible, to

- give priority to recommendations that extend Medicare solvency;[25] and
- give recommendations that
  - improve the health care delivery system and health outcomes, including by promoting integrated care, care coordination, prevention, and wellness, and quality and efficiency improvements;

- protect and improve Medicare beneficiaries' access to necessary and evidence-based items and services, including in rural and frontier areas;
- target reductions in Medicare program spending to sources of excess growth;
- consider the effects on Medicare beneficiaries of changes in payments to providers of services and supplies;
- consider the effects of recommendations on providers of services and suppliers with actual or projected negative cost margins or payment updates;
- consider the unique needs of Medicare beneficiaries who are dual-eligible for Medicare and Medicaid; and
- promote the delivery of efficient, high quality care to Medicare beneficiaries.

Content of Proposals

A proposal needs to include

- the Board's recommendations,
- an explanation of each recommendation and the reasons for including such recommendation,
- an actuarial opinion from the Chief Actuary certifying that the recommendations contained in the proposal:
  - will result in a net reduction in total Medicare program spending in the IY that is at least equal to the *applicable savings target*,[26] and
  - are not expected to result, over the ten-year period beginning with the IY, in any increase in the total amount of net Medicare program spending relative to what it would have been absent the proposal.

The Chief Actuary's certification in part restricts the Board from making recommendations that in the short term reduce spending but in the longer term (10 years), increase spending.

Therefore, Board recommendations may focus on[27]

- reductions in payments to Part C and Part D plans, including, among other things, direct subsidies to Part C and D plans and subsidies for non-Medicare benefits offered by Medicare Advantage plans;
- changes to payment rates or methodologies for services furnished in the fee-forservice sector by providers not otherwise addressed by changes such as competitive bidding or reductions in excess of productivity adjustments (see **Appendix C**); and
- changes that reduce costs by improving the health care delivery system and health outcomes.

Finally, after 2018, if the Chief Actuary projects that the *per capita rate of growth in national health expenditures* in the IY exceeds the projected *Medicare per capita growth rate* in the IY, then the Board's proposals need to be designed to help reduce the p*er capita rate of growth in national health expenditures* while maintaining or enhancing beneficiary access to quality care.

Exceptions to Developing Proposals

There are several circumstances when the Board will not need to transmit a proposal to Congress and the President. These are

- a year when the Chief Actuary determines that the *growth rate* does not exceed the *target growth rate*, or
- a year when the Chief Actuary determines that the projected percentage increase in the CPI_m in the IY is less than the projected percentage increase in the CPI_u.

Again, historically these circumstances have been rare. In addition, there are exceptions to implementing proposals which are discussed below.

OTHER BOARD RELATED ACTIVITIES

While the Board's principal function is to develop proposals that reduce per capita growth in Medicare spending, this is not its sole activity. The Board is charged with developing advisory reports related to Medicare, annual public information reports, and biennial reports containing recommendations to slow the growth in national health expenditures. Each type of report is detailed below, and a summary, with a timeline of the various Board reports, is presented in **Appendix A**. In addition, the Government Accountability Office (GAO) is directed, as described below, to undertake a review of the Board's initial recommendations and report to Congress by July 1, 2015.

Advisory Reports

Beginning January 15, 2014, the Board may develop and submit to Congress advisory reports on matters related to the Medicare program, regardless of whether or not the Board submits a proposal for such year. These advisory reports may include, for years prior to 2020, recommendations regarding improvements to payment systems for providers of services and suppliers who are not otherwise subject to the scope of the Board's recommendations (providers and suppliers scheduled to receive a reduction in their payment updates in excess of a reduction due to productivity [see **Appendix C**]).

Annual Public Reports

The Board will also produce an annual public report, beginning by July 1, 2014, that includes standardized system-wide information on health care costs, access to care, utilization, and quality of care that allows for comparison by region, types of services, types of providers, and both private payers and Medicare. [28]

Biennial Reports to Slow Growth in National Health Expenditures

Finally, in addition to Board proposals to control costs and the Board's annual public report, the Board will, beginning no later than January 15, 2015, and every two years thereafter, submit to Congress and the President recommendations to slow the growth in national health expenditures (excluding expenditures under this title and in other Federal health care programs) while preserving or enhancing quality of care. These recommendations are different from recommendations contained in any annual Board proposal and are not enacted by the Secretary unless Congress acts because the Board's official proposals can only include recommendations related to Medicare.[29] Rather, these recommendations can include matters that the Secretary or other federal agencies can implement administratively, matters that may require legislation to be enacted by Congress, matters that may require legislation to be enacted by state or local governments, or matters that can be voluntarily implemented by the private sector.

Consumer Advisory Council

The Board will be advised by a Consumer Advisory Council composed of 10 consumer representatives, appointed by the Comptroller General of the U.S. and from geographic regions established by the Secretary. The Consumer Advisory Council will meet no less frequently than twice a year, in Washington, DC, in public session. The law is silent on a date by which the Comptroller General needs to appoint the members of the Consumer Advisory Council and with respect to the term of service.[30]

Government Accountability Office Study

No later than July 1, 2015, the GAO is to submit a report to Congress containing the results of a study of changes to payment policies, methodologies, and rates and coverage policies and methodologies under the Medicare program as a result of the recommendations contained in the proposals made by the Board. The study is to include an analysis of the effects of Board recommendations on access, affordability, other sectors of the health care system, and quality of care. It may be the case that the impact of initial recommendations, if triggered in 2013, will not be fully ascertainable by July 1, 2015, thus making it difficult for GAO to analyze changes.

"FAST TRACK" PROCEDURES FOR CONGRESSIONAL CONSIDERATION

The Secretary must implement the Board's proposals unless Congress affirmatively acts to amend or block them within a stated period of time and under circumstances specified in the Act. As noted above, PPACA requires the Board to submit its proposal to both Congress and the President. The proposal is to be accompanied by, among other things, implementing legislation. The Secretary is required to automatically implement the proposals contained in the IPAB legislation on August 15 of the year such a proposal is submitted, unless

- prior to that date, legislation is enacted that includes the statement, "This Act supersedes the recommendations of the Board contained in the proposal submitted, in the year which includes the date of enactment of this Act, to Congress under section 1 899A of the Social Security Act," or
- in 2017, a joint resolution discontinuing the automatic IPAB implementation process has been enacted.[31]

To begin, § 3403(d) of the Act establishes special "fast track" parliamentary procedures governing House and Senate committee consideration, and Senate floor consideration, of legislation implementing the Board or Secretary's proposal. These procedures differ from the parliamentary mechanisms the chambers usually use to consider most legislation, and are designed to ensure that Congress can act promptly on the implementing legislation should it choose to do so. It accomplishes this goal by mandating the immediate introduction of the legislation in Congress, and by establishing strict deadlines for committee and Senate floor consideration, as well as by placing certain limits on the amending process. The procedures established by the Act permit Congress to amend the IPAB-implementing legislation, but only in a manner that achieves at least the same level of targeted reductions in Medicare spending growth as are contained in the IPAB plan. The Act bars Congress from changing the IPAB fiscal targets in any other legislation it considers as well, and establishes procedures whereby a super-majority vote is required in the Senate to waive this requirement.

The Act establishes a second set of "fast track" procedures governing the consideration of a joint resolution discontinuing the automatic IPAB implementation process described above. Such procedures are designed to promote timely consideration of such a joint resolution. This joint resolution requires a super-majority vote of both chambers and either the signature of the President or overriding his veto by a two-thirds vote in each house to enter into force.

Procedures for Considering IPAB-Implementing Bill

House and Senate Introduction of IPAB-Implementing Bill

On the day that the IPAB-implementing legislation is submitted to Congress by the President, it is to be introduced "by request" in each chamber by the House and Senate majority leaders or by a designee. [32] If a house is not in session on the day the proposal is submitted, the measure is to be introduced on the first day the chamber is in session thereafter. In the event that the House and Senate majority leaders fail to introduce the legislation within five days after the date on which the proposal is submitted to Congress (or after that chamber came into session after the proposal's submission), any Member may introduce the bill in his or her respective chamber.[33]

House and Senate Committee Referral, Report and Discharge

When introduced in the House, an implementing bill is to be referred to House Committees on Energy and Commerce and on Ways and Means. In the Senate, the measure is to be referred to the Committee on Finance. Not later than April 1 in any year in which a proposal is submitted, the three committees of referral may report the bill "with committee amendments related to the Medicare program." Rule XV of the Standing Rules of the Senate, which bars the Senate from considering a committee amendment containing any "significant matter" not in the jurisdiction of the committee recommending the amendment, does not apply to the IPAB legislation. The effect of the exemption is that the Committee on Finance may report committee amendments to the IPAB-implementing bill that include matter not in its jurisdiction "if that matter is relevant to a proposal contained" in the IPAB plan.[34]

If a committee of referral has not reported the IPAB-implementing bill to its respective chamber by April 1, the committee will be automatically discharged of further consideration of the legislation.

Congress Can Consider Only Legislation that Meets the Same Fiscal Targets as Those Recommended by the IPAB

The special parliamentary procedures established by the Act attempt to bar the House or Senate from considering any bill, resolution, amendment, or conference report pursuant to the special fast track procedures contained in the Act *or by any other legislative mechanism*, which would repeal or change the recommendations of the IPAB if that change would fail to achieve the same targeted reductions in Medicare spending growth achieved by the IPAB proposal. In other words, the procedures propose to bar Congress from considering, in any legislation (not just the IPABimplementing bill), changes to the Board's recommendations that fail to meet at least the same fiscal targets as those forwarded by IPAB. Because the Act establishes procedural rules related to congressional consideration not just of the IPAB-implementing bill, but also governing the consideration of other legislation as well, it differs from most expedited procedure statutes now in force.

The Act attempts to "entrench" this limitation on congressional action by stating that the provision can only be waived in the Senate by an affirmative vote of three-fifths of Senators chosen and sworn (60 votes if there is no more than one vacancy), the same threshold required to invoke cloture on most measures and matters. An appeal of a ruling on a point of order under this provision carries the same super-majority vote threshold to overturn the ruling of the Senate's presiding officer.[35]

Initial Senate Floor Consideration

The special parliamentary procedures established by the Act create an environment for Senate floor consideration of an IPAB-implementing bill which is similar to that which exists after the Senate has chosen to invoke cloture on a bill.

Under most parliamentary circumstances, a motion to proceed to consider legislation in the Senate is fully debatable.[36] Under the special procedures established by the Act, however, once an IPAB-implementing bill is on the Senate Calendar of Business, a non-debatable motion to proceed to its consideration is in order.[37] If the Senate chooses to take up the implementing bill by adopting this motion, consideration of the implementing legislation is limited to a total of 30 hours equally divided between the two party leaders, and a non-debatable motion to further limit debate is in order. This is a departure from Senate practice under its Standing Rules, during which debate on legislation is generally only limited by unanimous consent or by invoking cloture.[38]

Likewise, under the regular procedures of the Senate, debate on amendments is unlimited and there is no general requirement that amendments be germane.[39] Any amendments offered to the implementing bill in the Senate under the special procedures established by the Act, however, must be germane, and debate on each amendment is limited to one hour, equally divided between the bill manager and the offerer of the amendment. Debate on second-degree amendments, debatable motions, and appeals is limited to 30 minutes each, similarly divided.[40] The party leaders may yield time they control under the overall 30-hour cap to Senators during the consideration of any amendment, debatable motion, or appeal, should they choose to do so, however debate on any may not exceed 1 hour.

Not only must amendments be germane, but, as is noted above, the procedure established by the Act bars the consideration of any amendment (including committee amendment), which would cause the bill to result in a net reduction in the total Medicare program spending in the IY that is less than the applicable savings target established for that year and contained in the IPAB proposal. This limitation can only be waived by a vote of three-fifths of Senators chosen and sworn, and successfully appealing a point of order under this provision carries the same super- majority vote requirement.

After 30 hours of consideration, the Senate proceeds to vote on any pending amendments and then, once they are disposed of, on the measure itself, as amended, if amended. Prior to final passage, a motion to table or to reconsider is in order, as would be a demand for a live quorum call.

Initial House Floor Consideration

The Act does not establish fast track parliamentary procedures governing initial floor consideration of an IPAB-implementing bill in the U.S. House of Representatives. Should the House choose to act on such legislation, it would presumably do so under its usual procedures, most likely by adopting a special rule reported from the House Committee on Rules to establish terms for considering the bill.

Automatic "Hookup" of House and Senate Bill

The Act's special parliamentary procedures include provisions that are intended to facilitate the exchange of implementing legislation between the House and Senate.

First, the expedited procedures governing the Senate described above apply only to a bill received from the House if the same bill has been introduced in the Senate. In addition, the expedited procedures only apply in the Senate if the bill received from the House is related only to the programs under the Act and has satisfied the same fiscal targets as the IPAB-implementing bill. Such limitations are intended to prevent the special fast track procedures from being used to obtain expedited Senate consideration of unrelated legislation or legislative provisions.

The Act also establishes "hookup" procedures to ensure that the chambers will act on the same measure. If, before voting on its own implementing bill, a chamber receives an implementing bill passed by the other chamber, that engrossed legislation will automatically be amended by the text of the second chamber's bill and become the measure the receiving chamber votes on for final passage. If, after passing its own measure, a chamber receives an implementing bill passed by the other chamber, the vote on the receiving chamber's bill shall be considered to be the vote on the measure received from the other house as amended by the receiving chamber's implementing bill.

Consideration of a Conference Report or Amendment Exchange

The Act also establishes special parliamentary procedures for the expedited consideration of conference reports or amendments between the chambers intended to resolve bicameral differences on an IPAB-implementing bill. In either case, consideration of the IPABimplementing bill at the stage of resolving differences is limited by the Act to 10 hours of consideration in each chamber, equally divided between Senate party leaders, and in the House, between the Speaker of the House and its minority leader. Debate on any amendment under these procedures is limited to one hour and on second-degree amendments, motions, and appeals, to 30 minutes each. Here also, the expedited procedures apply only if the legislation is related only to the program under the Act and satisfies the same fiscal targets required of the IPAB bill.

Consideration of Veto Message

Should the President veto an IPAB-implementing bill, debate on the veto message in the Senate, which would under normal circumstances be unlimited, is confined to one hour, equally divided. There is no similar provision established for the House of Representatives, and it would presumably consider such a veto message under its regular parliamentary mechanisms.[41]

Procedures for Considering Joint Resolution Discontinuing the Independent Payment Advisory Board Process

Section 3403 of P.L. 111-148 establishes a second "fast track" parliamentary mechanism for consideration of legislation discontinuing the automatic implementation process for the recommendations of the Independent Payment Advisory Board described above.

Under the terms of the Act, in order to qualify for consideration under "fast track" procedures, a joint resolution discontinuing the process must meet several conditions:

- It must be introduced in 2017 by not later than February 1 of that year.
- It may not have a preamble.[42]
- It must have the title, "Joint resolution approving the discontinuation of the process for consideration and automatic implementation of the annual proposal of the Independent Medicare Advisory Board under section 1 899A of the Social Security Act."
- It must have the sole text, "That Congress approves the discontinuation of the process for consideration and automatic implementation of the annual proposal of the Independent Medicare Advisory Board under section 1 899A of the Social Security Act."

Introduction, Referral and Automatic Discharge

Under the terms of the Act, such a joint resolution may be introduced by any Member in either chamber. When introduced, the joint resolution is referred to the Committees on Ways and Means and on Energy and Commerce in the House, and to the Committee on Finance in the Senate.

In the Senate, if the Committee on Finance has not reported this joint resolution (or an identical joint resolution) by the end of 20 days of continuous session after its introduction, the committee may be discharged from its further consideration of the measure upon a petition signed by 30 Senators.[43] The committee could also mark up and report the joint resolution, although it is not required to do so, and if it does, it may not report amendments to it.

Senate Floor Consideration

At any time after a qualifying joint resolution has been placed on the Senate's Calendar of Business, it is in order to make a non-debatable motion to proceed to its consideration. Such a motion to proceed may be made even if one has been previously been rejected. As with the IPABimplementing bill procedure described above, the Act does not specify who may make this motion.

Points of order against the joint resolution and its consideration, with the exception of points of order established by the Congressional Budget Act of 1974 or any budget resolution enacted pursuant to the Budget Act, are waived.[44] If the Senate agrees to the motion to proceed, consideration of the legislation is "locked in"; the joint resolution remains the unfinished business of the Senate until it is disposed of.

Debate on a joint resolution discontinuing the automatic IPAB-implementing process and on all debatable motions and appeals in connection with the measure is limited to 10 hours in the Senate, with the time divided between the majority and minority leaders or their designees. A non-debatable motion to further limit debate is available.

No amendment (including committee amendment), motion to postpone, motion to proceed to the consideration of other business, or to recommit the joint resolution, may be made. At the conclusion of consideration, and after a single live quorum call, if requested, the Senate votes on the joint resolution. Passage of a joint resolution discontinuing the automatic IPAB process requires a supermajority of three-fifths of Senators, duly chosen and sworn.

House Floor Consideration

The Act does not establish special parliamentary procedures governing initial floor consideration of a joint resolution discontinuing the IPAB-implementing process in the House of Representatives. Should the House choose to act on such legislation, it would presumably do so under its regular procedures, most likely by adopting a special rule reported from the House Committee on Rules. Passage of the joint resolution in the House does, however, require a super- majority of three-fifths of Members, duly chosen and sworn, the same as in the Senate.

Automatic "Hookup" with other Chamber

As with the special procedures established for considering IPAB-implementing bills described above, the Act also establishes "hookup" procedures to facilitate the consideration in one chamber of a joint resolution passed by the other. If, before the passage by one house of a joint resolution discontinuing the IPAB-implementation process, that house receives an identical joint resolution from the other, that engrossed joint resolution will not be referred to committee, but will become the one on which the receiving chamber takes its final vote. Such provisions are designed to ensure that the House and Senate act on the same legislation.

Additional Considerations

Legislation May Face a High Bar
Both the implementing bill and the joint resolution described above are law-making forms of legislation, which must be signed by the President or enacted over his veto to become effective. Should either type of measure be vetoed by the President, overriding the veto would require a super-majority vote of two-thirds in both chambers for the measure to become law. The arguable and perhaps intended effect of the procedures in the Act is to favor the continuation of the IPAB and its recommendations even in the face of significant opposition in both chambers of Congress.[45] This is why some observers have argued that statutory disapproval mechanisms of the type contained in the Act shift the power balance to the executive branch and away from Congress.[46]

Either Chamber May Change the Parliamentary Procedure
The "fast track" parliamentary procedures established by the Act for the consideration of both types of IPAB legislation are considered to be rules of the respective houses of Congress even though they are codified in statute. As such, Congress has traditionally viewed them as subject to change in the same manner and to the same extent that any House or Senate rule can be altered by the Members of that chamber. In other words, Congress is not required to amend or repeal the statute to change the procedures. The House or Senate can change the procedures by unanimous consent, by suspension of the rules, or by special rule reported by the House Committee on Rules and adopted by the House.

Questions Exist about the Enforceability of the Procedures
As is described, above, the terms of the Act attempt to "entrench" the procedures themselves against change by requiring a super majority to amend them, as well as to discontinue the automatic IPAB-implementation process. The Act also purports to restrict the ability of future Congresses to enact certain policy changes related to Medicare in other legislation, not just the IPAB-implementing measure. How these entrenching provisions will be reconciled with the well- established constitutional right of each chamber of

Congress to make the rules of its own proceeding,[47] and how or if one Congress can broadly regulate the actions of a future Congress in this way, will likely only be clarified in practice.

Questions about the enforcement of these provisions are highlighted when one imagines how the consideration of IPAB legislation might play out in a future Congress. As has been noted, the House of Representatives normally brings major legislation to the floor under the terms of a special rule reported by its Committee on Rules. This is likely to be the method used by a future House of Representatives to consider IPAB-implementing legislation or other bill dealing with rates of Medicare spending.

Special rules establish unique terms for the consideration of legislation and routinely waive all points of order against the measure in question and its consideration. As such, it is unclear if there will be any parliamentary opportunity for a House Member to make a point of order against some future IPAB-implementing bill, for example, that the legislation violates the Act's stricture on changing targeted rates of Medicare spending. While one can certainly envision a Member making a rhetorical argument to that effect, a special rule which waives all points of order against such a bill and its consideration would effectively preclude enforcement of these terms of the Act. A "rider" discontinuing the automatic IPAB process entirely included in the conference report on an appropriations bill would similarly be unreachable by points of order if the report were considered under such a special rule or under the House's suspension of the rules procedure.

Questions about the enforcement of the Act's provisions similarly exist in the Senate. Traditionally, "fast track" procedures like those contained in the Act have been, in practice, more binding on the Senate than on the House, because the Senate views itself as a "continuing body" having rules that are continually in force. Additionally, altering such statutory procedures have arguably been more difficult in the Senate than in the House because to change its rules (including statutory rules) the Senate must effectively get all its Members to agree to waive them by unanimous consent or muster a super majority vote to suspend or amend them.

Unlike other statutory fast track procedures now in force, the Act establishes wide-ranging procedures which purport to regulate the consideration of not just one bill, but any legislation not meeting certain stated policy goals. To what extent a future Senate will view itself as bound by these broad terms, how the Senate's presiding officer will intelligently rule on certain points of order established by the Act, among other questions, will likely require additional clarification by the Senate.

IMPLEMENTATION OF BOARD MEDICARE PROPOSALS

In the absence of either one of the two general or one limited exceptions noted below, the Secretary implements the Board's proposals on August 15 of the PY. Essentially, recommendations that relate to payment rate changes that take effect on a fiscal year basis take effect on October 1 of the PY. Recommendations relating to payments to plans under Medicare Parts C and D and recommendations relating to payment rate changes that take effect on a calendar year basis take effect on January 1 of the IY.

There are two general exceptions to implementing a Board proposal:

1. If federal legislation was enacted by August 15 of the PY that superseded the Board's recommendations and
   a. achieves at least the same net reduction in total Medicare program spending as would have been achieved by the Board's proposal, and
   b. does not increase the expected Medicare program spending over the ten-year period, starting with the IY, relative to what it would have been absent the legislation.
2. Beginning with IY 2020, and beyond, the Secretary would not implement a Board proposal if a joint resolution was enacted prior to August 15, 2017, to discontinue the Board.

In addition, beginning in PY 2019, if the Board submitted a proposal in the prior year and in the current year the Chief Actuary determines that the projected *per capita rate of growth in national health expenditures* for the IY exceeds the projected *Medicare per capita growth rate* for the IY, then the Secretary is directed not to implement the recommendations submitted in the prior PY. For example, if in 2020 the Board submitted a proposal and in April 2021 the Chief Actuary determines that the projected *per capita rate of growth in national health expenditures* for 2023 exceeds the projected *Medicare per capita growth rate* for 2023, then the Secretary would not implement the recommendations contained in the 2020 proposal. However, the Secretary cannot use this exception in two successive years.

DISCUSSION AND POTENTIAL IMPACT OF IPAB

Qualifications and Recruitment of Board Members

By statute, the Board is to be composed of members drawn from a wide range of professions and backgrounds, in addition to geography, and a majority cannot be individuals directly involved in the provision or management of the delivery of Medicare items and services. What is not clear is whether this determination of a member's status is made at the time of nomination or whether a potential nominee's status is a function of their prior experience. For instance, would a retired executive from a Medicare Advantage plan be counted as being involved in the provision of Medicare services even though he or she may now be retired? Similarly, since there is a blanket prohibition on outside businesses, vocations, or employment, can a board member be characterized as an employer or being involved in the provision or management of services when he or she ceases employing anyone or ceases being involved in the provision of items or services?

One of the rationales for an independent board was to isolate health care payment decisions from the influence of special interests. While the statute specifies the qualifications of Board members, nationally recognized expertise, it also specifies that the Board should include, among others, employers, third-party payers, and representatives of consumers and the elderly. In moving beyond expertise, skills, and experience and naming specific groups that should be included on the Board, the legislation designates some interests as worthy of being represented and others, by omission, as not being worthy. These efforts, rather than isolating the Board from the influence of special interests appears to welcome some interests directly into the process. In addition, Board members, and the public more generally, may question whether certain Board members are on the Board in a representative capacity even though they are prohibited from outside businesses or employment.

While there is generally an adequate supply of individuals willing to serve on federal boards such as IPAB, the commitment (full time), modest salaries (relative to physicians, the private sector, and even some university appointments), and constraints on Board members (restrictions on outside employment and term of service) may make recruiting highly qualified and respected individuals problematic.[48] In addition, the prospect that Congress could pass a resolution to discontinue the Board only adds to this potential problem. Finally, while it does not appear that Board members reside locally, if this was a practical requirement for the operation of the Board, this could be an additional impediment.

Funding

The funding level for the Board as set forth in the legislation, and the size of the staff that could be supported by the funds, may constrain the Board's ability to develop more comprehensive recommendations to change payment mechanisms since such efforts are generally costly to design and test prior to implementation. While the Board's funding is slightly more than MedPAC's, the Board's charge is much broader than MedPAC's. In addition, since the Board is not responsible for administering the program, it will operate outside the Secretary's demonstration authority so will not be able, on its own, to experiment with and test new payment mechanisms. However, the Board may be able to effectively leverage its research capability and expand its capacity to focus on larger programmatic changes by working with MedPAC, the newly formed Center for Medicare and Medicaid Innovation, and CMS more generally. For instance, the Center for Medicare and Medicaid Innovation and the Board could coordinate in the design and testing of alternative payment models.

Savings over Time

CBO estimates cost savings from IPAB, during the 2015-2019 period, at $15.5 billion.[49] The Chief Actuary attributes savings of $24 billion due to IPAB through 2019.[50] The Chief Actuary warns that achieving growth rate targets in IYs 2015-2019 may be a "difficult challenge" given historic growth in per capita Medicare expenditures and the limitations on further reducing payments to providers and suppliers scheduled to receive a reduction in their payment updates in excess of a reduction due to productivity. In addition, the Chief Actuary points out that "after 2019, further Advisory Board recommendations for growth rate reductions would generally not be required if other savings provisions were permitted to continue."

Even if we assume that the Chief Actuary's estimate of savings is reasonable and achievable, total Medicare expenditures for the 2015 through 2019 period are forecast to be $3.9 trillion. The $24 billion in cumulative savings amounts to just slightly more that 0.6% of total program expenditures.

Put slightly differently, the projected savings from the Board's recommendations represent a reduction of $89.00 per year per Medicare beneficiary over the period 2015 through 2019.

Board Proposals

If the Board is to be fully successful it must balance both the short-term need to find savings with longer-term program and payment design issues. Changes that reduce costs by improving the health care delivery system and health outcomes often require several years before savings may occur and the Board may have to find immediate savings, therefore, Board proposals may skew toward changes in payments. To offset this potentiality, the Board may find it useful to work with the Center for Medicare and Medicaid Innovation to design and test demonstrations that may aid in longer term Board initiatives.

While the Board is charged with developing proposals that, in part, "target reductions in Medicare program spending to sources of excess growth," prior to 2019, the exemptions given to certain providers and suppliers of services or items that were subject to reductions in excess of a reduction due to productivity, means that other providers and suppliers will necessarily bear the brunt of any proposals prior to 2018. As noted earlier, these exempt providers represented roughly 37% of all Medicare benefit payments in 2009. While the argument for the exemption from Board proposals is that the exempt providers have already "taken a hit" by statutorily mandated changes in how their price adjustments are calculated, the consequence is that Board proposals can only target the remaining set of Medicare providers and suppliers. However, since total Medicare program spending is a function of both price and utilization, it is possible that some of the excess spending that potentially gives rise to the need for a Board proposal could be caused by increased payments to exempt providers and suppliers.

Impacts Beyond Medicare

While the Board's proposals can *only relate to the Medicare program*, the implications of its recommendations may have a much broader impact. Many payers fashion their payments on Medicare rates, such as "Medicare plus %," so recommendations to reduce Medicare payments for certain procedures or suppliers are likely to have a ripple effect throughout the health care system and could lead to a dampening of the average price paid for such services or supplies.

ACTIVITY RELATED TO IPAB DURING THE 112TH CONGRESS

Repeal Proposals

A number of bills have been introduced in the 112th Congress that would repeal PPACA completely. These include, among others, H.R. 2 and S. 192. Other bills have been introduced to amend the specific provisions of PPACA that relate to IPAB. For instance, H.R. 452, introduced by Representative Roe of Tennessee on January 26, 2011, would repeal PPACA §§ 3403 and 10320 (the IPAB provisions), including any amendments, and would restore any provisions of law amended by those sections. On March 29, 2011, Senator Cornyn introduced S. 668, the Health Care Bureaucrats Elimination Act, which would also repeal §§ 3403 and 10320 of PPACA.

The National Commission on Fiscal Responsibility and Reform

The National Commission on Fiscal Responsibility and Reform, popularly referred to as the Simpson-Bowles Deficit Commission, proposed two sets of recommendations (recommendations 3.5 and 3.6) regarding IPAB. Recommendation 3.5 proposed to "eliminate the provider carve-outs that exempt certain providers from any short-term changes in their payments (see **Appendix C**).[51] Recommendation 3.6 proposed to both establish "a global budget for total federal health care costs and limit the growth in federal health care spending to GDP plus 1%." The commission suggested that "expanding and strengthening the Independent Payment Advisory Board (IPAB) to allow it to make recommendations for cost-sharing and benefit design and to look beyond Medicare."

CBO March 2011 Baseline

On March 30, 2011, the CBO revised its estimate of the likely savings from IPAB. In testimony before the House Energy and Commerce Committee's Subcommittee on Health, CBO Director Douglas Elmendorf testified that:[52]

> In its February 2011 estimate, CBO concluded that the rate of increase in spending would probably exceed the target rate in some years, and that the IPAB, therefore, would have to intervene to reduce the growth of Medicare spending. CBO estimated that those actions would result in $14 billion in savings over the 2012–2021 period. In CBO's March 2011 baseline, by contrast, the rate of growth in Medicare spending per beneficiary is projected to remain below the levels at which the IPAB will be required to intervene to reduce Medicare spending. As a result of that reduction in projected Medicare spending, CBO's March baseline does not include any savings from actions by the IPAB.

While, this estimate may well change in the future with future changes in CBO's assumptions, CBO currently forecasts that IPAB will not generate any savings through 2021.

The President's April 13, 2011, Deficit Reduction Proposal

In President Obama's April 13, 2011, remarks on fiscal responsibility, the President called for

> strengthening an independent commission of doctors, nurses, medical experts and consumers ... to reduce unnecessary spending while protecting access to the services that seniors need. [And if] Medicare costs rise faster than we expect, then this approach will give the independent commission the authority to make additional savings by further improving Medicare.[53]

The President's proposal was further described in a fact sheet issued by the White House, which detailed that IPAB should target per beneficiary Medicare cost growth to GDP per capita plus 0.5% beginning in 2018 rather than the current 1%.[54]

Appendix A. Key Dates for IPAB Implementation

Table A-1. Effective Dates for § 3403 Provisions of PPACA

Requirement	Start or Effective Date or Deadline	End Date, Frequency or Duration
CY2013		
Chief Actuary of CMS submits determination of whether projected Medicare per capita growth rate for the implementation year (two years later) exceeds the projected Medicare per capita target growth rate for the implementation year; determination submitted annually thereafter.	4/30/2013	All subsequent years.
By this date, IPAB submits draft copy of proposal to the Secretary for review and comment, and to MedPAC for consideration.	9/1/2013	All subsequent years (subject to certain conditions).
CY2014		
Board is required to submit its first proposal to the President and Congress if the projected Medicare per capita growth rate for the implementation year exceeds the target growth rate for the implementation year. If the Medicare per capita growth rate does not exceed the target growth rate, the Board is required to submit an annual advisory report to Congress on matters related to the Medicare program.	1/15/2014	All subsequent years (subject to certain conditions).
If Board fails to submit proposal to Congress and the President, Secretary submits contingent proposal.	1/25/2014	Each subsequent year (subject to certain conditions).
Secretary submits report to Congress on results of review of Board's proposal (unless Secretary submits a proposal in that year). MedPAC submits comments to Congress on Board's proposal or the Secretary's proposal.	3/1/2014	All subsequent years (subject to certain conditions).
Deadline for specified Congressional Committees to consider the Board's proposal and report out legislative language implementing the recommendations. Congress has the authority to develop its own proposal provided it meets the same fiscal requirements as established for the Board.	4/1/2014	All subsequent years (subject to certain conditions).
Deadline for the Board to produce a public report containing standardized information on system-wide health care costs, patient access to care, utilization, and quality of care that allows for comparison by region, types of services, types of providers, and both private and public payers. Report is to be produced annually thereafter.	7/1/2014	All subsequent years.
Start date for the Secretary to begin implementing the Board's proposal. Any recommendation that would change a provider's payment rate will apply to items and services furnished on the first day of the first fiscal year, calendar year, or rate year (which varies depending on provider type) that begins after August 15.	8/15/2014	Each subsequent year (subject to certain conditions).

Table A-1. (Continued)

Requirement	Start or Effective Date or Deadline	End Date, Frequency or Duration
CY2015		
Deadline for the Board to submit to Congress and the President advisory recommendations to slow the rate of growth in national health expenditures. These recommendations could not target expenditures in federal health care programs. Recommendations are required at a minimum once every two years.	1/15/2015	At least once every 2 years thereafter.
Due date for GAO report on changes to payment policies, methodologies, and rates resulting from the Board's recommendations.	7/1/2015	Periodically in subsequent years.
CY2017		
Deadline for Congress to introduce a joint resolution discontinuing the Board's activities.	2/1/2017	
Deadline for Congress to enact a joint resolution discontinuing the Board's activities.	8/15/2017	
CY2018		
Board is only required to submit proposals to the President and Congress for years in which the projected rate of growth in Medicare spending exceeds the Gross Domestic Product (GDP) plus 1.0%.	1/15/2018	All subsequent years.
CY2019		
The first year the Board may begin submitting proposals that may reduce payments to providers and suppliers scheduled to receive a reduction in their payment updates in excess of a reduction due to productivity. These proposals would take effect in 2020.	1/15/2019	All subsequent years.

Source: CRS Report R41196, *Medicare Provisions in the Patient Protection and Affordable Care Act (PPACA): Summary and Timeline*, coordinated by Patricia A. Davis.

APPENDIX B. A COMPARISON OF IPAB AND MEDPAC

Table B-1. How Does IPAB Contrast to MedPAC

	IPAB	MedPAC
Located in	Executive Branch	Legislative Branch
Established under	Patient Protection and Affordable Care Act (PPACA, P.L. 111-148, § 3403).	Balanced Budget Act of 1997 (P.L. 105-33, § 4022) – by merging Prospective Payment Assessment Commission (ProPAC) and the Physician Payment Review Commission (PPRC)

	IPAB	MedPAC
Located in	Executive Branch	Legislative Branch
Principal Statutory Mandate	Make recommendations to be implemented by the Secretary of Health and Human Services to reduce the per capita rate of growth in Medicare spending; develop recommendations to slow the growth in national health expenditures while preserving or enhancing quality of care	Advise Congress on payments to private health plans participating in Medicare and providers in Medicare's traditional fee-for-service program; analyze access to care, quality of care, and other issues affecting Medicare
Authority	Board delegated significant policy making authority by Congress	Advisory
Size	15 appointed and 3 ex officio members	15 appointed members
Term	6-year term, staggered	3-year term, staggered
Appointed by	President in consultation with the majority leader of the Senate, the Speaker of the House of Representatives, the minority leader of the Senate and the minority leader of the House of Representatives	Comptroller General
Conditions of Employment	Full time, subject to ethical disclosures, compensation is level II (Chairperson) and level III (members) of the Executive Schedule, members may not engage in other business, vocation, or employment	Part time, subject to ethical disclosures, compensation is level IV of the Executive Schedule (with physician Commissioners receiving a comparability allowance)
Staff	Executive director and a staff to be determined	Executive director and a full time staff of 40
Powers and Work Product	Power to hold hearings and obtain official data Annual proposals, as required, annual and biennial reports	Power to obtain official data Public meetings and two annual reports
Budget	$15 million in FY2012 updated by the rate of inflation annually	$13 million in FY2011

Source: CRS analysis.

APPENDIX C. MEDICARE PRODUCTIVITY EXEMPTIONS AND BOARD RECOMMENDATIONS

PPACA § 3401 altered certain market basket updates used to adjust Medicare base payment amounts and incorporated productivity improvements into those market basket updates that previously did not include them. Since some providers and suppliers of services will receive a reduction in payments beyond their productivity adjustment in some years, Section 3403(c)(2)(iii) prohibits, as described below, the Board from recommending in some years further reduction in payment rates to those providers and suppliers.

All of the providers and suppliers subject to § 3401 productivity adjustments are listed in **Table C-1**. To be exempt under § 3403(c)(2)(iii) from Board recommendations in any given year a provider would have to be slated to receive a reduction under § 3401 in its inflationary payment update in excess of a reduction due to productivity in a year in which such recommendations would take effect.[55]

Reduction in Excess of a Reduction due to Productivity Adjustment

An "update reduction in excess of a reduction due to productivity" means that for that category of provider, after calculating any applicable percentage increase in payments due to changes in costs, reduced by the productivity adjustment, payments are further reduced by an additional applicable percentage specified in § 3401. For example, in rate year 2012, payments to long term care hospitals will be adjusted by changes in their costs, changes in productivity in the broader economy, and then reduced by an additional 0.10 percentage point. Again, only those providers that are subject to this additional reduction in payments will receive a time-limited exemption from Board recommendations.[56]

Table C-1. Providers of Services or Supplies Enumerated in § 3401

Applicable Exemptions, If Any, Under § 3403(c)(2)(iii)			
Providers of Services or Supplies	Inflationary Payment Update	Applicable Period[a]	Exemption Period[b]
Inpatient Acute Hospitals	Productivity adjustment Reduction in excess of a reduction due to productivity	Begins FY2012 FY2010-FY2019	Through 12/31/2019
Skilled Nursing Facilities	Productivity adjustment	Begins FY2012	None
Long-term Care Hospitals	Productivity adjustment Reduction in excess of a reduction due to productivity	Begins RY2012 RY2010-RY2019	Through 12/31/2019

Applicable Exemptions, If Any, Under § 3403(c)(2)(iii)			
Providers of Services or Supplies	Inflationary Payment Update	Applicable Period[a]	Exemption Period[b]
Inpatient Rehabilitation Facilities	Productivity adjustment Reduction in excess of a reduction due to productivity	Begins FY2012 FY2010-FY2019	Through 12/31/2019
Home Health Agencies	Productivity adjustment; Annual reduction of 1 percent	Begins CY2015; CY2011-CY2013	None
Psychiatric Hospitals	Productivity adjustment Reduction in excess of a reduction due to productivity	Begins RY2012 RY2010-RY2019	Through 12/31/2019
Hospice Care	Productivity adjustment Reduction in excess of a reduction due to productivity	Begins FY2013 FY2013-FY2019	Through 12/31/2019
Dialysis	Productivity adjustment	Begins CY2012	None
Outpatient Hospitals	Productivity adjustment	Begins CY2012	Through 12/31/2019
	Reduction in excess of a reduction due to productivity	CY2010-CY2019	
Ambulance Services	Productivity adjustment	Begins CY2011	None
Ambulatory Surgical Center Services	Productivity adjustment	Begins CY2011	None
Laboratory Services	Productivity adjustment Reduction in excess of a reduction due to productivity	Begins CY2011 CY2011-CY2015	Through 12/31/2015
Certain Durable Medical Equipment	Productivity adjustment	Begins CY2011	None
Prosthetic Devices, Orthotics, and Prosthetics	Productivity adjustment	Begins CY2011	None
Other Items	Productivity adjustment	Begins CY2011	None

Source: CRS analysis of P.L. 111-148, as amended. Notes:

a. FY = Fiscal Year; RY = Rate Year; CY = Calendar Year.

b. Since the first year the Chief Actuary in the Centers for Medicare & Medicaid Services can potentially make a determination that projected Medicare expenditures exceed the projected target is 2013, the earliest that any Board recommendations could be implemented would be August 15, 2014 for the fiscal year beginning in October. Therefore, exemptions are only potentially significant for the period beginning October 1, 2014 through December 31, 2019.

Therefore, the relevant factor in determining whether providers have an exemption is whether the provider had a reduction in excess of a reduction due to productivity in the year the recommendation would take effect. If so, that provider is exempt from Board recommendations that take effect in that year.

Providers Subject to § 3401

Table C-1 also indicates which providers are subject to a productivity adjustment, a reduction in excess of a reduction due to productivity, or some other adjustment; the applicable time period of the adjustment; and whether the adjustment gives rise to an exemption period under § 3403. CRS analysis of CMS statistics indicates that in 2009 Medicare payments to exempt providers represented approximately 37% of all Medicare benefit payments.[57]

Proposals generated by the Board in 2018 and submitted to the President and Congress in 2019 could include provisions, relating to any provider, that the Secretary would begin implementing effective August 15, 2019 and later. By 2020, all exemptions will have lapsed and all providers of services and supplies will potentially be subject to Board recommendations.

End Notes

[1] Section 3403(b). For a discussion of the Board and other new entities created pursuant to PPACA, see CRS Report R413 15, *New Entities Created Pursuant to the Patient Protection and Affordable Care Act*, by Curtis W. Copeland.

[2] As measured by the Bureau of Labor Statistics (BLS) U.S. city average all-items and U.S. city average medical care indices, http://www.bls.gov/data/#prices. As the BLS notes in Measuring Price Change for Medical Care in the CPI, http://www.bls.gov/cpi/cpifact4.htm, the CPI-medical care index only measures out-of-pocket consumer expenditures, including any health insurance premium amounts deducted through payroll withholdings. While this measure is commonly used to denote medical inflation, it measures changes in prices in only part of the health care system and may not be a good indicator of overall medical inflation or the growth in spending for medical care.

[3] Executive Office of the President, *Budget of the United States Government: FY2009, Historical Tables*, U.S. Government Printing Office, Washington, DC, 2008, pp. 26-27, http://www.gpoaccess.gov/usbudget/fy09/pdf/hist.pdf.

[4] This estimate is based on the growth in Medicare Parts A and B only and does not include the additional costs associated with Medicare Part D, coverage for prescription drugs, which was introduced in 2006. The Boards of Trustees, Federal Hospital Insurance and Federal Supplementary Medical Insurance Trust Funds, *2010 Annual Report of the Boards of Trustees of the Federal Hospital Insurance and Federal Supplementary Medical Insurance Trust Funds*, Washington, DC, August 5, 2010, p. 228.

[5] U.S. Department of Labor, Bureau of Labor Statistics, http://data.bls.gov/cgi-bin/cpicalc.pl. The Boards of Trustees, Federal Hospital Insurance and Federal Supplementary Medical Insurance Trust Funds, *2010 Annual Report of the Boards of Trustees of the Federal Hospital Insurance and Federal Supplementary Medical Insurance Trust Funds*, Washington, DC, August 5, 2010, p. 228.

[6] The Boards of Trustees, Federal Hospital Insurance and Federal Supplementary Medical Insurance Trust Funds, 2010 Annual Report of the Boards of Trustees of the Federal Hospital Insurance and Federal Supplementary Medical Insurance Trust Funds, Washington, DC, August 5, 2010, pp. 25, 33, and 228.

[7] U.S. General Accounting Office, *Health Care: Unsustainable Trends*, GAO-04-793SP, May 2004, p. 3, http://www.gao.gov/new.items/d04793sp.pdf.

[8] http://industry

[9] Tom Daschle, Scott S. Greenberger, and Jeanne M. Lambrew, *Critical: What Can We Do About the Health-care Crisis* (St. Martin's Press, 2008).

[10] Phillip Roe, "A Board Congress should nail," *The Washington Times*, July 23, 2010, http://www.washingtontimes.com/news/2010/jul/23/a-board-congress

[11] See § 3403(g)(1).

[12] See Department of Justice Memorandum entitled "Officers Of The United States Within The Meaning Of The Appointments Clause" for a discussion of why Board members can exercise the authority delegated to them under the statute. http://www.justice.gov/olc/2007/appointmentsclausev10.pdf.

[13] See § 3403(g)(2).

[14] See § 3403(g)(1)(C).

[15] See § 3403(g)(1)(D).

[16] See § 3403(g)(4).

[17] See §3403(l)(4).

[18] The average percentage increase over time is calculated using a geometric mean, which is the [nth root of the (value at the end of the time period divided by the value at the beginning of the time period)] − 1. A geometric mean is generally preferred to the arithmetic mean when measuring growth rates.

[19] For determination years after 2017, the *target growth rate* is the projected five-year average percentage increase, ending with the implementation year, in the nominal gross domestic product per capita plus one percentage point.

[20] This $3 billion savings target compares to $10.02 billion ([4.99%-3.32%] multiplied by $600 billion)—the amount projected spending exceeded targeted growth in spending. Again, in later years, different applicable percentage values are used and in any year if the projected excess in spending is less than the applicable savings target, then the projected excess for the implementation year (expressed as a percent) is the applicable percent.

[21] Richard S. Foster, Chief Actuary, Centers for Medicare & Medicaid Services, "Estimated Financial Effects of the "Patient Protection and Affordable Care Act", as amended" press release, April 22, 2010, http://burgess.house.gov/ UploadedFiles/4-22-2010_-_OACT_Memorandum_on_Financial_Impact_of_PPACA_as_Enacted.pdf.

[22] Direct subsidy payments are payments made by CMS on behalf of insureds, for cost-sharing elements of the benefit design with respect to low-income enrollees who are exempted by CMS from paying these elements themselves.

[23] The national average monthly bid amount is the average of the standardized bid amounts for each part D prescription drug plan and it is used to calculate the base beneficiary premium. Denying or removing high bids would lower the national average monthly bid amount.

[24] Medicare Part C and D plans may have been emphasized as a result of concerns regarding the higher costs of Medicare Advantage relative to Medicare fee-for-service, and unfavorable reports of some of their practices. "The average Medicare payment to Medicare Advantage plans is 113% of the cost of similar benefits in the original fee-forservice program." The Henry J. Kaiser Family Foundation, *Medicare at a Glance: Factsheet*, Washington, DC,

November 2008, http://www.kff.org/medicare/upload/1066_11.pdf. Also see U.S. Congress, House Committee on Energy and Commerce, Subcommittee on Health, *Profits, Marketing, and Corporate Expenses in the Medicare Advantage Market*, committee print, prepared by Committee Majority Staff, 111th Cong., 2nd sess., December 2009. However, the higher estimated spending under Part C relative to traditional Medicare may be reduced due to payment rate changes in PPACA.

[25] Medicare solvency generally refers to the Medicare Hospital Insurance (HI) Trust Fund since the Supplementary Medical Insurance (SMI) Trust Fund is currently adequately financed by the automatic financing structure established for Medicare Parts B and D. What is not clear from PPACA is to what extent the Board should favor Medicare Part A solvency over other parts of the Medicare program.

[26] In calculating the reduction in Medicare spending, the Chief Actuary is directed to count any reduction in spending achieved between October and December of a proposal year to the extent that such reductions were the result of the Secretary implementing, beginning October 1 of the proposal year, Board recommendations to change the payment rate for items or services.

[27] See PPACA § 3403(c)(2)(iv) and http://www.cbo.gov/ftpdocs/108xx/doc10868/12-19- Reid_Letter_Managers_Correction_Noted.pdf, p. 11.

[28] Since some of these topics touch closely on subjects that MedPAC has dealt with in the past, and to avoid unnecessary confusion between IPAB and MedPAC, refer to **Appendix B**, which highlights some of the differences between the two entities.

[29] § 3403(c)(2)(A)(vi).

[30] In addition, the Board is to regularly consult with the Medicaid and CHIP Payment and Access Commission created by the Children's health Insurance Program Reauthorization Act of 2009.

[31] Such a joint resolution and the procedures for its consideration are described later in this report.

[32] The term "by request" indicates that the measure is being introduced as a courtesy to the President, who can not introduce legislation, and that the sponsor of the bill does not necessarily favor it.

[33] Several existing expedited procedure statutes contain provisions for the mandatory introduction of legislation by House and/or Senate leaders. CRS is unaware of any instance in which a House or Senate officer failed to introduce legislation by request when directed to do so by such a statutory rule. For examples of such statutes, see U.S. Congress, House, *Constitution, Jefferson's Manual, and Rules of the House of Representatives*, H.Doc. 110-162, 1 10th Cong., 2nd sess. (Washington: GPO, 2009), §1130.

[34] Unlike germaneness, any requirement that amendments be "relevant" does not stem from Senate rules. It is a limitation that is traditionally only imposed on the amendment process by unanimous consent. In cases in which such a requirement has been imposed by unanimous consent, it has traditionally meant that the subject of an amendment must relate to the subject of the text it proposes to amend, and does not contain any significant subject matter not addressed by that underlying text.

[35] While, as is described elsewhere in this report, the Chief Actuary of the Centers for Medicare and Medicaid Services is to determine whether the IPAB proposal meets certain fiscal targets laid out by the Act, it is not specified how such a determination is to be made for other legislation Congress considers. How the Senate's presiding officer, for example, might rule on a point of order alleging that a given bill or amendment considered under regular parliamentary mechanisms violates this provision, is unclear. This question would likely require additional clarification by the Senate, no doubt made after close consultation with its Parliamentarian.

[36] A motion to proceed to consider is non-debatable in the Senate under certain limited circumstances, including under specific procedural statutes such as the Congressional Budget Act, when made during the Morning Hour, and when dealing with Executive Business and conference reports.

[37] The Act does not specify who can make the motion to proceed, and under the chamber's Standing Rules, any Senator may in theory lodge such a motion. By long-standing practice, however, Senators almost always defer to the majority leader or his designee to make such scheduling motions.

[38] For more information on cloture, see CRS Report 98-425, *Invoking Cloture in the Senate*, by Christopher M. Davis.

[39] The germaneness of amendments is required when amendments are offered to general appropriations bills, under some statutory rules (such as the Congressional Budget Act of 1974), to any legislation considered post-cloture, and when Senators agree to such a requirement by unanimous consent. Although the time for debate on amendments is unlimited in most circumstances, a non-debatable motion to table an amendment is in order in the Senate, and the effect of adopting such a motion would be to kill the amendment.

[40] If the bill manager favors the amendment, motion, or appeal, then the time in opposition will be controlled by the Senate minority leader or his designee.

[41] See CRS Report RS22654, *Veto Override Procedure in the House and Senate*, by Elizabeth Rybicki.

[42] A preamble is a series of "whereas" clauses at the beginning of a measure describing the reasons for and intent of the legislation.

[43] Days of continuous session are calculated by counting every calendar day, including Saturdays and Sundays, and pausing the count only at times when either chamber has adjourned for more than three days pursuant to a concurrent adjournment resolution.

[44] It is unclear if this wide-ranging waiver would prevent points of order under the Act itself from being raised against the joint resolution, for example, if it did not have the required text or has been amended.

[45] As of the date of this memo, the constitutionality of the Board is being challenged in *Coons v. Geithner,* a case filed by the Goldwater Institute in federal district court in Arizona. See http://www.goldwaterinstitute.org/CoonsvGeithner6. The three other current major challenges to PPACA, the Florida challenge (Florida v. HHS, No. 3:10-cv-91-RV/EMT (N.D. Fla., 2010), the Virginia challenge (Virginia ex rel. Cuccinelli v. Sebelius, No. 3:10cv188 (E.D. Va., 2010)), and the Thomas More Law Center challenge (Thomas More Law Ctr. v. Obama, (E.D. Mich, 2010)) did not raise constitutional objections to IPAB. For a discussion of some of the constitutionality issues see CRS Report R40725, *Requiring Individuals to Obtain Health Insurance: A Constitutional Analysis*, by Jennifer Staman et al.. In Baldwin v. Sebelius, No. 10-1033, (S.D. Cal., 2010), dismissed by the trial court, but under appeal, also did not challenge IPAB. There is always the possibility of future constitutional challenges to the Board once it is constituted and takes an action.

[46] See, for example, Rep. Claude D. Pepper, remarks in the House, *Congressional Record*, vol. 134, July 7, 1988, p. 17071.

[47] U.S. Constitution, Article I, sec. 5.

[48] Timothy Stolzfus Jost, "The Independent Payment Advisory Board," *The New England Journal of Medicine*, vol. 363, no. 2 (July 8, 2010), pp. 103-105; http://www.cq.com/display.do?dockey=/cqonline/prod/data/docs/html/weeklyreport/111/weeklyreport111-000003636595.html@allnews&metapub=CQ-WEEKLYREPORT&searchIndex=0&seqNum=15&productId=5.

[49] Letter from Douglas W. Elmendorf, Director, Congressional Budget Office, to Honorable Nancy Pelosi, Speaker, House of Representatives, March 20, 2010, http://www.cbo.gov/ftpdocs/113xx/doc11379/AmendReconProp.pdf.

[50] Richard S. Foster, Chief Actuary, Centers for Medicare & Medicaid Services, "Estimated Financial Effects of the "Patient Protection and Affordable Care Act", as amended" press release, April 22, 2010, http://burgess.house.gov/ UploadedFiles/4-22-2010_-_OACT_Memorandum_on_Financial_Impact_of_PPACA_as_Enacted.pdf.

[51] The complete commission report can be found at http://www.fiscalcommission.gov/sites/fiscalcommission.gov/files/documents/TheMomentofTruth12_1_2010.pdf.

[52] Douglas W. Elmendorf, *CBO's Analysis of the Major Health Care Legislation Enacted in March 2010*, Congressional Budget Office, Washington, DC, March 3, 2011, http://www.cbo.gov/ftpdocs/121xx/doc12119/03-30- HealthCareLegislation.pdf.

[53] The President's full remarks can be found at http://www.whitehouse.gov/the-press-office/2011/04/13/remarkspresident-fiscal-policy

[54] http://www.whitehouse.gov/the-press-office/2011/04/13/fact-sheet-presidents-framework-shared-prosperity-

[55] Some Medicare providers are paid according to fee schedules that are updated on an annual basis to reflect changes in their costs. Under prior law these annual updates did not include an adjustment for changes in the productivity of Medicare providers. Beginning in 2012, PPACA reduces the annual update to some providers by a productivity adjustment equal to the 10-year moving average of changes in annual economy-wide private nonfarm multifactor productivity. See CRS Report RL3 0526, *Medicare Payment Policies*, coordinated by Paulette C. Morgan for a general discussion of Medicare payment policies.

[56] See CRS Report R41 196, Medicare Provisions in the Patient Protection and Affordable Care Act (PPACA): Summary and Timeline, coordinated by Patricia A. Davis, **Appendix B**, for a timeline of update reductions and productivity adjustments, by provider.

[57] U.S. Department of Health and Human Services, *2009 CMS Statistics*, Centers for Medicare & Medicaid Services, Baltimore, MD, August 2009.

In: Medicare Spending and the Independent ... ISBN: 978-1- 62081-112-2
Editors: R. D. Brown and S. J. Martin © 2012 Nova Science Publishers, Inc.

Chapter 2

PPACA: A BRIEF OVERVIEW OF THE LAW, IMPLEMENTATION, AND LEGAL CHALLENGES[*]

Hinda Chaikind, Curtis W. Copeland, C. Stephen Redhead and Jennifer Staman

SUMMARY

In March 2010, the 111th Congress passed health reform legislation, the Patient Protection and Affordable Care Act (P.L. 111-148), as amended by the Health Care and Education Reconciliation Act of 2010 (P.L. 111-152). Jointly referred to as PPACA, the law increases access to health insurance coverage, expands federal private health insurance market requirements, and requires the creation of health insurance exchanges to provide individuals and small employers with access to insurance. The costs for expanding access to health insurance and other provisions are projected to be offset by increased taxes and revenues and reduced Medicare and Medicaid spending. Implementation of PPACA, which is scheduled to unfold over the next few years, involves all the major health care stakeholders, including the federal and state governments, as well as employers, insurers, and health care providers. Following the enactment of PPACA, state attorneys general and others have brought a number of

---

[*] This is an edited, reformatted and augmented version of a Congressional Research Service publication, CRS Report for Congress R41664, from www.crs.gov, dated March 2, 2011.

lawsuits challenging provisions of PPACA, including the individual mandate, on constitutional grounds.

This report provides a brief summary of major PPACA provisions, implementation and oversight activities, and current legal challenges.

INTRODUCTION

The 111th Congress passed major health reform legislation, the Patient Protection and Affordable Care Act (P.L. 111-148), which was amended by the Health Care and Education Reconciliation Act of 2010 (P.L. 111-152). Jointly, these laws are referred to as PPACA. This report provides a brief summary of major PPACA provisions, implementation and oversight activities, and current legal challenges.

OVERVIEW OF HEALTH REFORM LAW

PPACA increases access to health insurance coverage, expands federal private health insurance market requirements, and requires the creation of health insurance exchanges to provide individuals and small employers with access to insurance. PPACA increases access to health insurance coverage by expanding Medicaid eligibility, extending funding for the Children's Health Insurance Program (CHIP), and subsidizing private insurance premiums and cost-sharing for certain lower-income individuals enrolled in exchange plans, among other provisions. These costs are projected to be offset by increased taxes and other revenues and reduced Medicare and Medicaid spending. The law also includes measures designed to enhance delivery and quality of care.

While most of the major provisions of the law do not take effect until 2014, some provisions are already in place, with others to be phased in over the next few years.

Coverage Expansions and Market Reforms: Pre-2014

The law creates several temporary programs to increase access and funding for targeted groups. They include (1) temporary high-risk pools for uninsured individuals with preexisting conditions; (2) a reinsurance program to reimburse employers for a portion of the health insurance claims' costs for their 55- to 64-year-old retirees; and (3) small business tax credits for firms with fewer than 25 full-time equivalents (FTEs) and average wages below $50,000 that choose to offer health insurance. Additionally, prior to 2014, states may choose to voluntarily expand their Medicaid programs.

Some private health insurance market reforms also take effect prior to 2014, such as extending coverage to children up to age 26 and not allowing children up to age 19 to be denied insurance and benefits based on a preexisting condition. Major medical plans can no longer impose any lifetime dollar limits on essential benefits, and plans may only restrict annual dollar limits to defined amounts. Plans must cover preventive care with no cost-sharing, and they cannot rescind coverage, except for fraud. They must also establish an appeals process for coverage and claims. Insurers must also limit the ratio of premiums spent on administrative costs compared to medical costs, referred to as medical loss ratios, or MLRs.[1]

Coverage Expansions and Market Reforms: Beginning in 2014

The major expansion and reform provisions in PPACA take effect in 2014. State Medicaid programs will be required to expand coverage to all eligible non-pregnant, non-elderly legal residents with incomes up to 133% of the federal poverty level (FPL). The federal government will initially cover all the costs for this group, with the federal matching percentage phased down to 90% of the costs by 2020. The law requires states to maintain the current CHIP structure through FY2019, and provides federal CHIP appropriations through FY2015 (thus providing a two-year extension on CHIP funding).[2]

States are expected to establish health insurance exchanges that provide access to private health insurance plans with standardized benefit and cost-sharing packages for eligible individuals and small employers. In 2017, states may allow larger employers to purchase health insurance through the exchanges, but are not required to do so. The Secretary of Health and Human Services (HHS) will establish exchanges in states that do not create their own approved exchange. Premium credits and cost-sharing subsidies will be available to individuals who enroll in exchange plans, provided their income is generally above 100% and no more than 400% of the FPL and they meet other requirements.

Also beginning in 2014, most individuals will be required to have insurance or pay a penalty (an individual mandate). Certain employers with more than 50 employees who do not offer health insurance may be subject to penalties. While most of these employers who offer health insurance will meet the law's requirements, some may be required to also pay a penalty if any of their full-time workers enroll in exchange plans and receive premium subsidies.

PPACA's federal health insurance requirements are further expanded in 2014, with no annual dollar limits allowed on essential health benefits and no exclusions for preexisting conditions allowed regardless of age. Plans offered within the exchanges and certain other plans must also meet essential benefit standards, covering services such as emergency services, hospital care, physician services, preventive services, prescription drugs, and mental health and substance use disorder services, among others. Premiums may vary by limited amounts, but only based on age, family size, geographic area, and tobacco use. Additionally, plans must sell and renew policies to all individuals and may not discriminate based on health status.

Health Care Quality and Payment Incentives

PPACA contains a number of provisions to create and/or study payment incentives and service delivery models that are designed to improve quality of health and health care and to reduce expenditures. The law establishes pilot, demonstration, and grant programs to test integrated models of care, including accountable care organizations (ACOs), medical homes that provide coordinated care for high-need individuals, and bundling payments for acute-care episodes (including hospitalization and follow-up care). PPACA establishes the Center for Medicare and Medicaid Innovation, to pilot payment and service delivery models, primarily for Medicare and Medicaid beneficiaries. The law also establishes new pay-for-reporting and pay-for-performance programs within Medicare that will pay providers based on the reporting of, or performance on, selected quality measures.

Additionally, PPACA creates incentives for promoting primary care and prevention, for example, by increasing primary care payment rates under Medicare and Medicaid; covering some preventive services without cost-sharing; and funding community-based prevention and employer wellness programs, among other things. In addition, the law increases funding for community health centers and the National Health Service Corps to expand access to primary care services in rural and medically underserved areas and reduce health disparities. PPACA also requires the Secretary of Health and

Human Services (HHS) to develop a national strategy for health care quality to improve care delivery, patient outcomes, and population health.

Cost Containment and Financing of Health Reform

The Congressional Budget Office (CBO) and the staff of the Joint Committee on Taxation (JCT) estimated the direct spending and revenue effects of PPACA.[3] CBO projects that PPACA will reduce federal deficits by $143 billion over the 10-year period of 2010-2019 and, by 2019, will insure 94% of the non-elderly, legally present U.S. population.

The costs of the coverage expansions under the law are offset by provisions designed to (1) slow the rate of growth of federal health care spending and (2) increase revenues through taxes and penalties.[4] PPACA incorporates numerous Medicare payment provisions to slow the rate of growth in federal health care costs, including reductions in Medicare Advantage (MA) plan payments and a lowering of the annual payment update for hospitals and certain other providers.[5] PPACA also establishes an Independent Payment Advisory Board (IPAB) to make recommendations for achieving specific Medicare spending reductions if costs exceed a target growth rate. IPAB's recommendations will take effect unless Congress overrides them, in which case Congress would be responsible for achieving the same level of savings. Finally, PPACA provides tools to help reduce fraud, waste, and abuse in both Medicare and Medicaid.

PPACA increases revenue using several mechanisms. Individuals who do not have health insurance, as well as large employers who do not comply with the law's requirements to provide such insurance, may be subject to penalties. PPACA raises a large share of its revenue from taxes on high-income households, such as an additional Medicare payroll tax on those with incomes over $200,000 (single) and $250,000 (married). PPACA also creates an excise tax on high-cost plans. The law limits the annual contribution to Flexible Spending Accounts (FSAs) to $2,500, and excludes over-the-counter medications (except insulin) from reimbursement by FSAs and other health tax savings accounts.

In calculating its estimates of the cost and savings of PPACA, CBO projected that the law will reduce the number of uninsured by 32 million people, leaving 23 million residents uninsured by 2019. Those without coverage will include those who choose not to purchase health insurance and are subject to the penalty for non-compliance and those who are exempt from the individual mandate for religious or other reasons, as well as about 7-8 million illegal immigrants.

IMPLEMENTATION AND OVERSIGHT

Implementation of PPACA, which is scheduled to unfold over the next few years, involves all the major health care stakeholders, including the federal and state governments, as well as employers, insurers, and health care providers. While the HHS Secretary is responsible for implementation and oversight of many of PPACA's provisions, other federal officials and entities are also given new responsibilities. For many of the law's most significant reform provisions, the Secretary is required to take certain actions (e.g., promulgate regulations) by a specific date. As already noted, many of the key components of market reform and coverage expansion do not take effect until 2014. Implementing some parts of the law will entail extensive rulemaking and other actions by federal agencies; other changes will be largely self-executing, pursuant to the new statutory requirements. PPACA also creates a variety of new commissions and advisory bodies, some with substantial decision making authority (e.g., IPAB).

States must expand Medicaid coverage and are expected to take the lead in establishing the exchanges, even as many of them struggle with budget shortfalls and weak economies. Employers, too, have a key role to play in PPACA implementation. The law makes changes to the employer-based system under which millions of Americans get health insurance coverage. Many small employers will face decisions on whether to use the new incentives to provide coverage to their employees, while larger employers must weigh the benefits and costs of continuing to offer coverage or paying the penalties for not doing so.

The federal subsidies and outlays for expanding insurance coverage represent mandatory spending under the new law. In addition, PPACA appropriates and transfers from the Medicare trust funds billions of dollars over the coming years to support many of the law's provisions. They include providing funding for states to plan and establish exchanges (once established, exchanges must become self-sustaining), and support for a center to test innovative payment and service delivery models. PPACA creates three multi-billion dollar trust funds to support health centers and health workforce programs, comparative effectiveness research, and public health programs. Finally, the law authorizes funding for numerous new and existing discretionary grant programs. Obtaining funds for such programs and activities requires action by congressional appropriators.

Rulemaking

PPACA is being implemented in a variety of ways, including new agency programs, grants, demonstration projects, guidance documents, and regulations. Of these, only regulations have the force of law and can compel action by non-federal individuals and organizations. The federal rulemaking process is governed by the Administrative Procedure Act (APA, 5 U.S.C. §551 et seq.), other statutes, and executive orders, with agencies generally required to publish proposed rules, take comments from the public, and then publish a final rule. Agencies' compliance with the APA is subject to judicial review. More than 40 provisions in PPACA require or permit agencies to issue rules, with some allowing the agencies to "prescribe such regulations as may be necessary." As of December 2010, federal agencies had issued about 20 final rules to implement the legislation, and indicated that they planned to issue more than three dozen proposed and final rules in 2011.[6]

Congressional Oversight

Congress has a range of options as it oversees the implementation of PPACA, including oversight hearings, confirmation hearings for agency officials, letters to and meetings with agency officials, and commenting on proposed or final rules. Congress, committees, and individual Members can also request that the Government Accountability Office or federal agency inspectors general evaluate agencies' actions to implement PPACA. The Congressional Review Act (5 U.S.C. §801 et seq.) requires that all final rules be submitted to Congress before they can take effect, and provides expedited procedures (primarily in the Senate) by which Congress can disapprove agencies' rules. A congressional resolution of disapproval must be signed by the President for it to take effect. Congress can also include provisions in the text of agencies' appropriations bills directing or preventing the development or enforcement of particular regulations.

LEGAL CHALLENGES

Following enactment of PPACA, state attorneys general and others have brought a number of lawsuits challenging provisions of PPACA, including the individual mandate, on constitutional grounds. For example, in *Florida v. HHS*, attorneys general and governors in 26 states as well as others have brought an action against the Secretaries of Health and Human Services, the Treasury, and Labor, seeking relief from the individual mandate and other PPACA requirements. In *Virginia ex rel. Cuccinelli v. Sebelius*, the Virginia attorney general filed a separate lawsuit challenging the federal requirement to purchase health insurance. Many expect that one or more of these cases will reach the Supreme Court.[7]

Constitutional Issues

At issue in many of the lawsuits is whether Congress has the authority to pass the individual mandate under either its power to regulate interstate commerce or its taxing power. Under the Commerce Clause, one issue is whether the requirement to purchase health insurance is a valid regulation of economic activity or an unconstitutional attempt to regulate inactivity. Supporters argue that the requirement to purchase health insurance is economic in nature because it regulates how an individual participates in the health care market, through insurance or otherwise. Opponents contend that while regulation of the health insurance industry or the health care system is economic activity, requiring the purchase of health insurance is not economic regulation. While supporters emphasize that requiring Americans to have health insurance is important for the proper functioning of the U.S. health care system, opponents stress that requiring a private individual to purchase health insurance would be an unprecedented expansion of Congress' commerce powers.

Supporters of the individual mandate also argue that Congress can use its taxing powers to encourage taxpayers to purchase health insurance. Opponents assert that since the tax associated with the individual mandate may be avoided by purchasing insurance, it is a penalty and thus the taxing power does not, by itself, provide Congress the constitutional authority to support this provision.

States' Rights Issues

The states and the federal government have a very complicated, shared power relationship when it comes to health care. Recently, this relationship has engendered intense and contentious debate, with considerable resistance by a number of states in the form of lawsuits, statutes, and constitutional amendments intended to limit, opt-out of, or nullify certain PPACA provisions, most often the individual mandate.[8]

Legislation attempting to nullify selected provisions of PPACA has been enacted in several states. In addition, voters in some states recently approved state constitutional amendments intended to keep the purchase of health insurance optional for individuals. If the underlying constitutional issues are resolved by the courts in favor of Congress's power to enact the individual insurance mandate, then these state nullification provisions would likely be ineffective under the Supremacy Clause of the U.S. Constitution, under which federal laws are the "supreme Law of the Land."[9]

End Notes

[1] For more information on the private health insurance provisions in PPACA, see CRS Report R40942, *Private Health Insurance Provisions in the Patient Protection and Affordable Care Act (PPACA)*, by Hinda Chaikind, Bernadette Fernandez, and Mark Newsom.

[2] For more information about the Medicaid provisions in PPACA, see CRS Report R41210, *Medicaid and the State Children's Health Insurance Program (CHIP) Provisions in PPACA: Summary and Timeline*, coordinated by Julie Stone.

[3] CBO's and JCT's final estimate of PPACA dated March 20, 2010, includes the provisions in both, P.L. 111-148 and the amendments in P.L. 111-152. It is available at http://www.cbo.gov/ftpdocs/113xx/doc11379/AmendReconProp.pdf.

[4] For more information on the revenue provisions in PPACA, see CRS Report R41128, *Health-Related Revenue Provisions in the Patient Protection and Affordable Care Act (PPACA)*, by Janemarie Mulvey.

[5] For more information about the Medicare provisions in PPACA, see CRS Report R41196, *Medicare Provisions in the Patient Protection and Affordable Care Act (PPACA): Summary and Timeline*, coordinated by Patricia A. Davis.

[6] For more information about regulations in PPACA, see CRS Report R41586, *Upcoming Rules Pursuant to the Patient Protection and Affordable Care Act*, by Curtis W. Copeland and Maeve P. Carey, and CRS Report R41346, *Initial Final Rules Implementing the Patient Protection and Affordable Care Act*, by Curtis W. Copeland.

[7] For further analysis of the constitutionality of the individual mandate and a discussion of these lawsuits, see CRS Report R40725, *Requiring Individuals to Obtain Health Insurance: A Constitutional Analysis*, by Jennifer Staman et al.

[8] For a discussion of states' rights issues in the context of health care, see CRS Report R40846, *Health Care: Constitutional Rights and Legislative Powers*, by Kathleen S. Swendiman.
[9] U.S. Const. Art. VI, cl. 2.

INDEX

A

access, vii, viii, 2, 3, 17, 18, 19, 20, 21, 36, 37, 39, 47, 48, 49, 50
adjustment, 39, 40, 41, 42, 46
Administrative Procedure Act (APA), 53
age, 49, 50
agencies, 5, 9, 21, 52, 53
alters, 2
appointments, 7, 32
Appointments Clause, 43
appropriations, 30, 45, 49, 53
assessment, 8
authority, 5, 6, 10, 33, 36, 37, 39, 43, 52, 54, 62

B

base, 18, 39, 43, 50
beneficiaries, 4, 18, 50
benefits, viii, 2, 16, 19, 43, 49, 50, 52
board members, 8
bonuses, 17
budget resolution, 28
Bureau of Labor Statistics, 4, 42, 43
businesses, 32

C

certification, 18
challenges, viii, 45, 48
commerce, 54
community, 50
compensation, 39
competition, 5
compliance, 51, 53
conference, 24, 26, 30, 44
Conference Report, 26
conflict of interest, 9
Congress, vii, viii, 1, 2, 3, 6, 9, 10, 16, 19, 20, 21, 22, 23, 24, 27, 29, 30, 32, 35, 37, 38, 39, 42, 43, 44, 47, 48, 51, 53, 54, 55
Congressional Budget Act of 1974, 28, 45
Congressional Budget Office, 2, 5, 45, 46, 51
consent, 7, 24, 29, 30, 44, 45
Constitution, 7, 44, 45, 55
constitutional amendment, 55
constitutional challenges, 45
constitutional issues, 55
consumer expenditure, 42
Consumer Price Index (CPI), 4, 9, 11, 13, 42
consumers, 8, 32, 36
cost, vii, viii, 2, 3, 15, 16, 18, 33, 35, 36, 43, 48, 49, 50, 51
cost saving, 33

D

demonstrations, 34
Department of Health and Human Services, 9, 46
Department of Justice, 43
Department of Labor, 4, 43
disability, 9
disorder, 50
doctors, 36
draft, 6, 16, 37
drugs, 42, 50

E

economic activity, 54
economics, 8
emergency, 50
employees, 9, 49, 52
employers, viii, 8, 32, 47, 48, 49, 51, 52
employment, 9, 32, 39
enforcement, 30, 53
England, 45
environment, 24
executive branch, 6, 9, 29
executive orders, 53
expenditures, vii, 1, 2, 4, 5, 6, 7, 10, 11, 12, 13, 14, 16, 17, 19, 20, 21, 31, 33, 38, 39, 41, 42, 50
expertise, 5, 8, 32

F

federal agency, 53
federal government, 49, 55
federal law, 55
federal private health insurance market requirements, viii, 47, 48
Federal Reserve Board, 5
financial, 5, 9
force, 2, 23, 24, 30, 53
formula, 6, 12
fraud, 49, 51
funding, 7, 17, 33, 48, 49, 50, 52, 53

funds, 9, 33, 52, 53

G

GAO, 20, 21, 38, 43
GDP, 11, 12, 13, 35, 36, 38
GDP per capita, 12, 13, 36
General Accounting Office, 43
geography, 32
governments, viii, 21, 47, 52
grant programs, 50, 53
grants, 53
gross domestic product, 43
Gross Domestic Product, 11, 38
growth, vii, 1, 2, 3, 4, 5, 6, 7, 11, 12, 13, 14, 15, 16, 17, 18, 19, 21, 22, 24, 31, 33, 34, 35, 36, 37, 38, 39, 42, 43, 51
growth rate, vii, 1, 6, 7, 11, 12, 13, 14, 15, 16, 17, 19, 31, 33, 37, 43, 51
guidance, 53

H

health, vii, viii, 3, 5, 6, 8, 17, 19, 20, 21, 31, 32, 34, 35, 37, 38, 39, 42, 44, 47, 48, 49, 50, 51, 52, 53, 54, 55, 56
Health and Human Services (HHS), vii, 1, 3, 7, 9, 39, 45, 46, 49, 51, 52, 54 health care, vii, viii, 3, 5, 6, 17, 19, 20, 21, 32, 34, 35, 37, 38, 42, 47, 50, 51, 52, 54, 55, 56
health care costs, 20, 35, 37, 51
health care programs, 5, 21, 38
health care system, 21, 34, 42, 54
health expenditure, 17, 19, 20, 21, 31, 38, 39
health insurance, viii, 42, 47, 48, 49, 50, 51, 52, 54, 55
health insurance exchanges, viii, 47, 48, 49
health services, 8
health status, 50
homes, 50
hospitalization, 50

Index

House, 2, 7, 22, 23, 24, 25, 26, 27, 28, 29, 30, 36, 39, 44, 45
House of Representatives, 7, 25, 26, 28, 30, 39, 44, 45

I

immigrants, 52
improvements, 5, 17, 20, 39
income, 43, 48, 49, 51
increase cost sharing, viii, 2
Independent Payment Advisory Board, 1, iii, v, vii, 1, 3, 6, 27, 35, 45, 51
individuals, viii, 7, 8, 32, 47, 48, 49, 50, 53, 55
industry, 43, 54
inflation, 3, 4, 11, 39, 42
inspectors, 53
insulin, 51
issues, 34, 39, 45, 55, 56

J

jurisdiction, 9, 23

K

kill, 45

L

laws, 48, 55
lead, 35, 52
leadership, 7
legislation, viii, 2, 5, 21, 22, 23, 24, 25, 26, 27, 28, 29, 30, 31, 32, 33, 44, 45, 47, 48, 53
lifetime, 49
lobbying, 9
local government, 21

M

major health care stakeholders, viii, 47, 52
majority, 7, 8, 17, 22, 23, 24, 25, 28, 29, 30, 32, 39, 45
malfeasance, 9
management, 8, 32
mark up, 27
Medicaid, vii, viii, 1, 2, 3, 18, 33, 34, 41, 43, 44, 45, 46, 47, 48, 49, 50, 51, 52, 55
medical, 3, 4, 11, 13, 36, 42, 49, 50
medical care, 13, 42
Medicare, 1, iii, vii, viii, 1, 2, 3, 4, 5, 6, 7, 8, 9, 10, 11, 12, 13, 14, 15, 16, 17, 18, 19, 20, 21, 22, 23, 24, 25, 27, 29, 30, 31, 32, 33, 34, 35, 36, 37, 38, 39, 41, 42, 43, 44, 45, 46, 47, 48, 50, 51, 52, 55
Medicare beneficiary, vii, 1, 4, 5, 16, 17, 34
Medicare program expenditures, vii, 1, 12, 16
membership, 7
mental health, 50
models, 33, 50, 52

N

naming, 32
National Health Service, 50
national strategy, 51
neglect, 9
New England, 45
nominee, 32
nurses, 36

O

Obama, 36, 45
Obama, President, 36
officials, 5, 6, 52, 53
omission, 32
operations, 7
oversight, viii, 48, 52, 53

P

parliamentary procedure, vii, 2, 3, 22, 24, 25, 26, 28, 29
Patient Protection and Affordable Care Act, vii, viii, 1, 3, 38, 42, 43, 45, 46, 47, 48, 55
payroll, 42, 51
penalties, 50, 51, 52
permission, iv
permit, 22, 53
physicians, 8, 32
policy, 5, 6, 29, 30, 39, 46
policy making, 39
policy reform, 6
pools, 48
population, 51
poverty, 49
power relations, 55
preparation, iv
prescription drugs, 42, 50
President, 2, 6, 7, 9, 10, 16, 19, 20, 22, 23, 26, 29, 36, 37, 38, 39, 42, 44, 46, 53
President Obama, 36
prevention, 17, 50
price index, 9
private sector, 21, 32
procedural rule, 24
Procedure in the House, 45
professionals, 8
prosperity, 46
public health, 5, 53
public opinion, 6

Q

qualifications, 32

R

raise premiums, viii, 2
ration care, viii, 2, 16

recommendations, 2, 5, 6, 10, 12, 15, 17, 18, 20, 21, 22, 24, 27, 29, 31, 33, 34, 35, 37, 38, 39, 40, 41, 42, 44, 51
recruiting, 32
reduced Medicare, viii, 47, 48
reform, vii, viii, 3, 5, 6, 47, 48, 49, 52
Reform, 5, 35, 48, 51
reforms, 6, 49
regulations, 52, 53, 55
regulatory changes, 15
reimburse, 48
reinsurance, 48
requirements, viii, 10, 37, 47, 48, 49, 50, 51, 52, 54
resolution, 22, 24, 27, 28, 29, 31, 32, 38, 44, 45, 53
restrictions, 32
revenue, 51, 55
rights, 56
risk, 48
root, 43
rules, 24, 29, 30, 44, 45, 53

S

savings, vii, 1, 3, 5, 6, 7, 12, 14, 16, 18, 25, 33, 34, 36, 43, 51
savings account, 51
science, 8
scope, 6, 20
Senate, 2, 6, 7, 22, 23, 24, 25, 26, 27, 28, 29, 30, 39, 44, 45, 53
services, 4, 8, 11, 18, 19, 20, 32, 34, 35, 36, 37, 39, 42, 44, 50
Social Security, 22, 27
spending, vii, viii, 1, 2, 3, 4, 5, 6, 7, 11, 12, 13, 14, 15, 18, 19, 22, 24, 25, 30, 31, 34, 35, 36, 38, 39, 42, 43, 44, 47, 48, 51, 52
stakeholders, viii, 47, 52
Standing Rules, 23, 24, 45
state, viii, 21, 47, 52, 54, 55
states, 49, 52, 54, 55, 56
statistics, 42
statutes, 24, 44, 53, 55
structure, vii, 3, 7, 44, 49

Index

subsidy, 17, 43
substance use, 50
suppliers, 2, 16, 18, 20, 33, 34, 38, 39, 40
Supreme Court, 54
sustainable growth, 6

T

target, vii, 1, 7, 10, 11, 12, 13, 14, 15, 16, 18, 19, 25, 34, 36, 37, 38, 41, 43, 51
tax credits, 49
taxes, viii, 47, 48, 51
taxpayers, 54
technology, 8
testing, 33
tobacco, 50
Treasury, 54
trial, 45
triggers, viii, 2, 7
trust fund, 9, 52
Trust Fund, 9, 42, 43, 44

U

U.S. Department of Labor, 4, 43
uninsured, 48, 51

United States, 7, 42, 43

V

veto, 23, 26, 29
vote, 17, 22, 23, 24, 25, 26, 29, 30
voters, 55
voting, 26

W

wages, 49
waiver, 45
Washington, 21, 42, 43, 44, 46
waste, 51
wellness, 17, 50
White House, 36
workers, 50
workforce, 52

Y

yield, 25